Coping Courageously

Praise for Coping Courageously

"Coping Courageously is an essential guide for families facing serious illness. With insight and compassion, Dr. Chiaramonte offers a lifeline for those struggling to manage the emotional, physical, and spiritual impact of illness. Drawing on the principles of integrative medicine and palliative care, Dr. Chiaramonte provides practical tools for reducing uncertainty, managing overwhelm, and finding greater peace and resilience at a difficult time. This powerful book offers hope and healing, reminding us that even in the face of illness, we can still find moments of beauty, connection, and profound meaning. A must-read for anyone seeking to navigate the challenges of serious illness with grace and dignity."

Andrew Weil, MD
Founder and Director, Andrew Weil Center for Integrative Medicine
Lovell-Jones Endowed Chair in Integrative Medicine

"Dr. Chiaramonte brilliantly weaves her personal and professional journeys to teach us how to address the most significant life challenges. She provides us with the necessary tools to have difficult conversations but gives us the space to be with our messy emotions . . . finding strength in our vulnerability."

Darshan Mehta, MD, MPH
Medical Director, Benson-Henry Institute for Mind Body Medicine
Assistant Professor of Medicine, Harvard Medical School
Education Director, Osher Center for Integrative Medicine

"As an integrative medicine physician, I am always in search of compassionate and practical resources for families facing serious illness. Dr. Delia Chiaramonte's book, *Coping Courageously: A Heart-Centered Guide for Navigating a Loved One's Illness Without Losing Yourself,* is a remarkable and transformative guide that stands out in this field.

Dr. Chiaramonte's extensive experience as an integrative palliative medicine physician and educator is evident in her powerful stories and invaluable insights. This book is not just a guide, but a lifeline for families navigating the complex emotional and physical challenges of illness. With its holistic approach to tackling vital topics often overlooked in traditional medical settings, *Coping Courageously* is an essential resource for families in need of guidance, support, and wisdom. I wholeheartedly endorse it."

Melinda Ring, MD
Executive Director, Osher Center for Integrative Health at Northwestern University

"Dr. Chiaramonte tells the story of families navigating the toughest journey that they have ever had to take—intentionally, mindfully moving through serious illness. She does so with the empathetic lens of a caring and skilled physician, offering skills-based tools and guided questions that help both patients and their loved ones face the reality of mortality courageously. Her sensitivity working with each family helped them muster what they needed—to successfully navigate the road before them. I am filled with gratitude for the number of patients and families that will utilize this work of hope, a roadmap for making the most important journey of all."

Maryanna Klatt, PhD
Director of Integrative Health,
The Ohio State University College of Medicine

"Drawing on her personal and considerable clinical experience, Dr. Chiaramonte has written the book we all need to weather the storm of a loved-one's serious illness. Powerful, relatable anecdotes and practical guidance combine to make this book compelling and so useful for supporting your loved one, navigating complex health care environments, and caring for yourself so you can better care for your family member. No one should suffer the suffering of others without the help of this marvelous, indispensable book."

Mark Komrad, MD
Psychiatrist and Medical Ethicist
Johns Hopkins University School of Medicine

"Dr. Chiaramonte's book, *Coping Courageously*, is the first practical and honest guide for caregivers and families of seriously ill patients. Caring for a loved one with serious illness can lead to exhaustion, confusion and feelings of failure. *Coping Courageously* provides practical guidelines, reassurance, and comfort to caregivers and families trying to navigate this delicate time. I highly recommend this book to all patients, families, as well as, medical professionals during this most challenging time in one's life."

Patricia Attman, MD
Psychiatrist
University of Maryland School of Medicine

A Heart-Centered Guide
for Navigating a
Loved One's Illness
Without Losing Yourself

Coping Courageously

Delia Chiaramonte, MD, MS

Published by Insight Health Publishing

ISBN (paperback): 979-8-9897999-0-9
ISBN (ebook): 979-8-9897999-1-6

Book design and production by www.AuthorSuccess.com

Printed in the United States of America

All patient names have been changed to protect their privacy. Some stories include composites of several patients.

This book does not provide medical advice, and nothing in it should be considered medical care, medical advice, or a doctor-patient relationship.

Dedication

This book is dedicated to my husband and daughters who support me without question whenever I have a crazy idea for a project, like writing a book, and to our beloved Coco, who unfailingly curled up beside me as I wrote and allowed me to practice what I preach. It is also lovingly dedicated to my cousin Steve, who made the theoretical real.

Free Offers

The Essential Caregiving Checklist: What You Need to Do If Someone You Love is Ill

If someone you love is sick, you may feel overwhelmed, exhausted, and unsure. There are so many details and things to worry about that it can be hard to know what to focus on. As an integrative palliative care physician who has cared for many families just like you, I've created a **practical checklist** to guide you.

This helpful guide provides key steps to help your family effectively navigate this challenging time.

You can find the free Essential Caregiving Checklist at:
www.CopingSupport.com

For Physicians and Clinicians:
How to Support Families Who Are Facing Serious Illness

If you are a physician, nurse practitioner, physician assistant, social worker, chaplain, or other healthcare clinician, you want to support your patients or clients (and their families) as they face serious illness, but you may not know exactly what to say or how best to help.

As an integrative palliative care physician, I know just how tough this can be. I've created an **integrative symptom management guide** to help you deliver the best possible care to your seriously ill patients.

It includes effective and simple ways to care for yourself too, because if you get depleted you can't be the empathetic clinician that you want to be. If you're not at your best, nobody wins.

Expanding your toolbox to include an evidence-supported integrative approach is the best way to care for your patients, their families, and yourself.

Get your helpful clinician guide at:
www.CopingSupport.com

Contents

Introduction

Of course, it happened while I was on a business trip.

"She fell off a horse," my husband said on the phone, while I was in the car on the way to the hotel.

He had taken our twelve-year-old daughter to her horseback riding lesson and ten minutes into the lesson the horse had spooked. For no discernable reason, the horse suddenly took off, racing around the track with wide eyes and a single-minded plan to escape some imagined terror. No one could stop him. My sweet daughter was hanging on with all her strength. She was bouncing against his powerful flank as he ran, and my husband watched in horror as she slowly slid down the huge horse's body.

"JUST LET GO!" her instructor screamed.

She did, and she ended up on the ground, headfirst, with a dented helmet and a dented life trajectory.

My husband called me as they were driving home.

"She seems okay," he said. "I took her out for ice cream."

"Can I talk to her?" I asked him.

He handed her the phone.

"Hi," she said in a subdued voice. She didn't sound like herself.

"Hey bunny, what happened?" I asked.

"I don't know, Mama." I felt my stomach drop.

"What do you mean you don't know?" I asked.

"I can't remember anything. I just remember sitting on the ground against the fence, and my head really hurts," she said.

I tried to keep my voice light, "Can I talk to Daddy?"

I knew then that she had a concussion, but I had no idea about the dark cloud that was about to descend upon her and upon our family.

You'll read more of my daughter's story later, but here is what's important for now. She suffered profoundly, both physically and emotionally, for several years, and she, her sister, her father, and I were all deeply impacted by this experience. Her pain was unbearable, and her brain no longer worked the way she wanted it to. She felt intermittently furious and hopeless, and we felt impotent to make it better. The mood in the house became suffocating, and sometimes we felt like we were drowning.

It was a long few years.

The medical system alone failed to heal my daughter. And "healers" alone couldn't do it, either. We longed for a simple way out of this maze. Ultimately, working together as a family and exploring both conventional and unconventional healing traditions is what helped. The combination of medications, steroid injections, surgery, physical and psychological therapy, guided imagery, yoga, massage, aromatherapy, and finding meaning in her experience finally gave my daughter her life back.

We, her family, were part of her journey. Even when she was flailing and suffering and unsure of her future, she knew that she wasn't walking this painful road alone. We took turns making space for her pain so she didn't need to suffer in loneliness. We kept the flame of hope burning for when she couldn't imagine a way out of the darkness. We lifted her up when she couldn't keep going all by herself. This was tough, and caring for ourselves became a crucial part of caring for her. We needed to learn to radically attend to our own wellbeing so that our flame could keep burning. How could we help her climb out of the swirling dark hole that had engulfed her if we allowed our own light to extinguish? We were all stuck in this web together and we needed each other to break free.

I had seen in my work, and then in my life, that illness is a family affair. My two worlds, as a mom and as a physician, had coalesced and I had a feeling that something important would emerge from the brutal experience of dealing with my daughter's accident. Even though my husband and I are both physicians, we weren't able to locate a doctor to effectively guide us through the heartbreaking fallout of her head injury. We longed for someone who would see her as a whole person, understand the importance of caring for the entire family, and skillfully use the best of conventional and complementary treatments to relieve all of our suffering.

We were off course and needed a captain to steer our heaving ship back to safety. We never found one. Some of my daughter's physicians said we just needed to wait for her to get better, others told her the pain was all psychological, one steered us to a helpful procedure but had such a prickly bedside manner that we hesitated to take his advice, and another told her everything would get better if she just stopped eating sugar. We wanted an expert to use the best of science and healing arts to help her, and to help our whole family. Since we never found a guide, I became the guide.

This experience solidified my commitment to what I call "integrative palliative medicine." This fusion of two discrete person-centered specialties is exactly what families need when they are facing a complicated and distressing medical situation. The combination of integrative medicine and palliative medicine creates an approach to care that I describe as whole family care for people with serious illness, using all the tools that work. Integrative palliative medicine is not widely recognized, at least not yet, but it should be. This is my crusade.

Integrative medicine uses treatment modalities, called complementary therapies, such as massage, acupuncture, and mind-body approaches that are not standardly taught in medical schools. The belief that the mind and body are connected is fundamental to the field, and there is a general interest in using safer, less invasive tools before more aggressive ones when it is safe to do so. There are many studies published in scientific journals that show the benefits of complementary treatments, such as acupuncture to treat chemotherapy-induced nausea and meditation to treat pain.

Unfortunately, when the field was young it called itself "alternative medicine" and touted some unproven treatments, which gave many physicians a sour taste and has left a stain on the field that persists. Plenty of physicians tell their patients, inappropriately in my opinion, to "stop using all that unproven stuff." However, practitioners of complementary or integrative medicine can be equally judge-y in the opposite direction, advising their patients to avoid medications, procedures, and surgery in favor of raw diets, herbal supplements, or clearing mold from the basement.

Those in the extreme hang tightly to their opposing points of view, but there is plenty of space for the rest of us in the middle.

Palliative medicine is the whole-person care of people with serious illness and their families, focused on relieving suffering rather than curing disease. It is appropriate as soon as someone is diagnosed with a serious illness, even if the individual is hoping to be cured. Palliative care physicians and other team members, such as nurse practitioners, nurses, social workers, chaplains, home health aides, and volunteers help patients and families to relieve symptoms, cope with the stress of illness, and make treatment decisions. There is a great misconception, even among physicians, that palliative care is the same as hospice, and thus is only for people who are near the end of their life. This misguided myth robs people of the powerful gifts that palliative care can offer.

I believe diverse perspectives are not mutually exclusive. They can peacefully coexist. I believe that you can endure hardship and find meaning. I believe that you can find joyful moments even when someone that you love is ill. I believe that you can combine complementary treatments with conventional medical treatments to help people with serious illness and their families live their best possible lives. I believe that the burdens that you are carrying can be lightened, and I am passionate about helping you to lighten them.

I have seen the power and impact of this approach in action. For nearly a decade I was the associate director and director of education for the University of Maryland Medical School Center for Integrative Medicine. There I taught medical students and residents to skillfully use evidence-supported integrative medicine and I supervised an integrative medicine service for people sick enough to be admitted to the hospital. More recently, I created and led an integrative palliative medicine program at Greater Baltimore Medical Center/Gilchrist and served there as division chief of integrative palliative medicine. The program that I created brought both disciplines, integrative medicine and palliative medicine, together. The work was deep and meaningful. In addition to me, an integrative palliative medicine physician, our team included nurse practitioners, a social worker, a mind-body specialist, music therapists, and an acupuncturist. We all felt honored to be invited into families' lives at such a challenging time. We tried to relieve their stress and suffering, we laughed with them, we cried, we went to funerals, and I even went to one beautiful and touching wedding.

All the families in my practice faced diagnoses that you wouldn't want. They dealt with shock, terror, and grief for the people that they used to be before the doctor said, "I'm sorry to tell you this, but . . ."

By the way, my use of the word 'family' includes your chosen family, your soul family, your family of origin, and anyone else, human or otherwise, who is an important part of your world.

My patients bore the brunt of the burden. They endured nausea, fatigue, constipation, and pain. They got biopsied or dialyzed, sat in chemo chairs, or had surgery. They had pills to swallow and decisions to make. Yet it wasn't only my patients who were affected; they usually did not make this journey alone. When the patients cried and suffered, their loved ones cried and suffered, too. Facing the darkness made some people shrink and withdraw. Some raged. Others felt numb. But some people grew.

Over time, I saw the energy in some families shift. With openness, self-reflection, and the bravery to face the darkness, families transformed. They shucked all the stupid junk from their lives and focused on what, and who, brought them joy. They worked on keeping their minds in the present moment and making that moment as great as it could possibly be. They hung out together, went to the beach, played the guitar, drew pictures, sewed gowns, and painted rocks. They swallowed more pills than they wanted to so that they could feel well enough to fully live their lives. They golfed, and if the patient couldn't golf anymore, they rode in the golf cart as a family. This was integrative palliative medicine in action. It was powerful.

I don't mean to paint a Pollyanna picture. My patients also puked and cried and shaved off their hair before the chemo made it fall out in chunks. Their families grieved and bickered and ate too many donated lasagnas. The road was sometimes brutal, but sometimes it was sweet. Families healed old wounds that were stupid and not worth being mad about anymore. Clutter got thrown out, clearing space for meditation corners.

These families weren't, for the most part, grateful for the illness, and they didn't think "everything happens for a reason." But what they did do is look for the flowers that fought their way out of the rocks. And what they found were stronger relationships, new perspectives, and time away from regular responsibilities. This allowed them to take a breath, spend time at their loved one's bedside, and read some of those books on the nightstand. They learned to shift their gaze away from the toughest of the tough stuff until their flowers came into view.

I learned so much from these perfectly imperfect people. And what I learned from them, I'm going to share with you. When you shift your gaze away from your heaviest burdens and fears, can you see a hint of flowers?

This book has three parts.

Part I is about navigating the experience of illness and taking bold and impactful action. In this section, you will learn how to help your special person find their own flowers, maintain their sense of self, and make tough medical decisions based on their unique goals. You will also find guidance for dealing successfully with the medical system and getting the best possible care for your loved one.

Part II is about cultivating growth and resilience. You will learn how to balance your caring and your life, and how to fill up your own cup so you have the energy and empathy to care for your loved one without losing yourself.

Part III is about strengthening authentic and meaningful connections. In this section you will learn how to handle family conflict, have tough conversations with your loved ones, manage anticipatory grief, and gather together to review the touching, meaningful, and funny moments of your family life.

In each section you will find exercises, thought-provoking questions to discuss with family and friends, and practical tools to lighten your burden.

After reading this book you will gain:

- The confidence to know that you are helping your loved one in the best way you can

- Tools and techniques to reduce the distress level of everyone in the family

- Peace of mind even when your loved one's illness can't be cured

Let's face it—life can be hard.

We have little control over the burdens that life sends our way. Relationships will sour, people we love will get sick, and we'll face losses of many kinds. This book can't fix any of that, and you cannot avoid emotional pain and sadness.

Yet with courage and knowledge, what you *can* do is extremely powerful. This book is your guide.

PART I

Navigate Challenges and Take Bold Action

CHAPTER 1

Find Flowers in the Poop

I keep a compost container on my kitchen counter. I fill it with apple cores and strawberry tops, with the papery thin membranes that cover my garlic, and the seeds from sliced up red peppers. I add coffee grounds and banana peels. It looks like trash.

I take it outside, open our big green barrel, shoo away the swarm of tiny bugs, and dump the mess inside. Months later, after baking in the sun, my nasty, smelly garbage has turned to soft, dark brown, nutrient-rich soil.

The plants in my yard are grateful for this trash-turned-soil and for the manure that the landscapers bring each spring. They thrive because of the nitrogen, phosphorus, and other nutrients that they pull from the garbage.

The poop helps my flowers to grow.

You are probably dealing with a large amount of metaphorical poop right now. Either you're ill, or someone that you care about is ill, or you take care of people who are ill. Either way, there is almost certainly a lot of poop on your path, and you are probably doing your best to avoid stepping in it as you navigate this challenging time.

Even when there is poop everywhere you look, there might be a tiny flower peeking its head out of the smelly mess and stretching itself toward the sun.

The stories that you're about to read are about me, but they are also about you. The hard parts of life don't spare any of us. Life is a mixed bag of tough stuff, happy stuff, and lots of grocery shopping and taking the dog to the vet. It's easy to take the happy times for granted, and common to be utterly shocked when life takes a tough turn. Our response to the painful, hurtful, scary, or sad parts of life is almost always to do whatever we can to get the heck out of that situation ASAP. Yet sometimes escape isn't an option. You may not be able to control every situation, but you *can* control which parts of the situation you focus on. You can focus on the sadness or on the increased time together. On the fear or on the sweetness of looking through photo albums as a family. On the frustration of a cranky loved one or on the closer sibling relationship that has grown out of caring for an ill parent together. The tough times can have sweet moments, and sometimes good things grow out of bad ones.

Sometimes "flowers" grow from "poop."

Story #1

Poop

When I was little, I used to call Dial-A-Joke for company. I was an only child and a latchkey kid, and my single mother didn't enjoy mothering. In retrospect, I can see that she was depressed, but at the time I simply knew that she didn't seem to like me very much and life didn't feel calm or safe.

The soundtrack of my childhood was my mother screaming, "I'M GOING TO F*CKING KILL MYSELF BECAUSE OF YOU!!"

I heard it if I cried or lost five dollars or couldn't find my shoes. I heard it at home, on the streets of Manhattan, and in the supermarket.

I heard it so often that I can hear it still. And since she did, in fact, try to kill herself, I believed her.

When I was nine years old, one of her boyfriends offered to take nude photos of me and another threatened to shoot me. One night, my mother screamed, "Delia, help me!" when one of these unsavory guys had her pinned up against the wall in our apartment with his fist in the air.

I came running and he said, in a terrifyingly quiet voice, "Get the f*ck back to your room or I'll kill you."

I scurried back to my room and felt overwhelming guilt as I quietly closed my bedroom door. She wasn't wounded that day, but I was.

I was brutally shy and, although I did well in school, I didn't have many friends. I didn't have much guidance growing up and I never found a supportive adult to fill in for my absent mother. She moved out when I was sixteen, leaving me to live alone in our apartment. She paid the rent, but I was left to figure out complex young adult issues, including the college application process, on my own. I only applied to one school, with a rank far below what I could have achieved, and it was a terrible fit. I didn't visit until move in day and I was shocked, when I showed up in my flowy skirt and Birkenstocks, to find a sea of cowboy hats and pointy boots.

I chose a college major, French literature, that I have never used and had a huge career crisis in my senior year. After messing up schedules and prerequisites, I ended up two years behind my peers and I didn't get into my first-choice medical school. I chose a specialty (family medicine) that I no longer practice, and I make significantly less money than many of my physician peers. While my friends have spent decades in the same practice, I have held a bunch of different jobs, never quite finding a perfect place to land.

My husband works all the time, so I don't see him much. We rarely go out and my friends have joked that they're not even sure I'm married because I always show up to events alone. Both of my children have had significant health issues, which put a huge emotional strain on the family. There were times, for each of them, when I wasn't sure they would ever be okay.

What an *unlucky* person I am.

Now I'm going to tell you another story.

Story #2

Flowers

My mother had untreated depression and didn't love parenting, but I never worried about being hungry or homeless. There were some challenging times, like when I came home from sleepaway camp at age eleven, shocked to find our apartment all packed up. Word on the street was that my mother's ex-boyfriend had been released from prison and was planning to kill her, and me, for her role in getting him locked up. While I was making lanyards and getting mosquito bites, my mother arranged for us to move across the country. Off we went to Los Angeles to start a new life.

My new L.A. school was a gem, and it unquestionably changed my life. This school, The Area D Alternative School, was created by New Age parents seeking a unique think tank-type of learning environment. I became me because of that school. If we hadn't had to leave New York, I might never have blossomed into the person that I am.

My first job, at age twelve, was scooping poop at a dog kennel. I saved my money and planned the type of grownup that I would be. I decided that I could either fall apart or become strong enough to take care of myself. The strength that I chose has become woven into the fabric of who I am. It has led me to opportunities and insights that I might have missed if I had been born into a softer world.

When I graduated early from high school at age seventeen, I bought a plane ticket, backpack, and Eurail pass, and planned a solo adventure abroad.

When my mother asked, "What if I say you can't go?" I laughed.

"It's too late for that," I said, and off I went to spend four months traveling Europe on my own.

It was a life-changing experience.

People hadn't always shown up for me, but animals had, so I had planned to be a veterinarian. I picked a university with a great vet school, but I didn't bother to visit before I showed up for classes. When I drove up to the school in my little white Toyota packed with everything I owned, I felt like I'd entered a foreign and exciting world. Everyone looked so different from anyone that I had known. I didn't find *MY* people, but I did find some people and I had a lot of fun. I went dancing, drank wine in a hot tub in the snow, tried skiing, and read *Camus* in French. I studied abroad in Paris and worked for a veterinarian. At the last minute, I changed my career plans and applied to medical school. Even though this new plan set me back a couple of years, I am grateful for that life-altering fork in the road.

If I had stayed in Colorado, I would never have met my devoted husband or had my two cherished daughters. My supportive and caring husband works a lot, but his dedication to providing for his family allowed me to work part-time when our children were young. I will always be grateful to him for giving me that time with our daughters. I may not have risen to the pinnacle of my career, but I did attend field trips, career day, and every school show. I couldn't be happier with the trade-off.

I didn't expect to love mothering, so I was surprised when my heart ballooned at the birth of each of my children. From the moment I became one, I have adored being a mommy. Since I didn't have strong motherhood modeling, I read and observed and self-reflected and healed my wounds so I could show up for my daughters as the mother they needed.

When each of my girls faced their own significant health challenges, I gathered my strength to walk beside them and advocate for their recovery.

I helped them find meaning in their experiences and sat next to them when they dissolved in tears of hopelessness or fear. We all fell down from time to time, but each time we got up again. My husband and I each carried our own part of the burden, and we never turned against each other.

I am humbled to see the wise, kind, resilient, and generally fabulous young women that my daughters have become. My husband and I are adjusting to our empty nest.

What a *lucky* person I am.

Do you get it?

We each have poop stories and flower stories. Every moment of every experience, no matter how challenging, can be seen through poop glasses or flower glasses. We get to choose which glasses we put on.

Don't get me wrong, I'm not suggesting that you should feel grateful that your loved one is ill. I'm sure you would give anything to make them well. Hard things are hard and imposing toxic positivity doesn't make them less hard. Yet, in each moment, we get to choose where we focus our attention. If we focus on all the negative dimensions of this moment or this experience, we feel worse. It's as simple as that. If we acknowledge the negative parts, but then shift our attention to some of the sweet or powerful or meaningful parts, we can find slivers of growth and inspiration and hope.

We can find flowers in the poop.

Remember my daughter's tumble from a horse? The only thing she remembers is feeling certain that she was going to die.

What followed that accident was several years of hell. For her, for me, for her dad, and for her sister. We all suffered in different ways, but she undoubtedly suffered the most. Her unbearable headaches started by the time she got home from the barn after her fall and didn't lift, even for a moment, for almost a year. She went to bed with excruciating pain, lay awake for hours contemplating how her life had fallen apart, and woke with no relief at all. Everything about her life had changed, and none of it had changed for the better.

We started to see the world as BC (before concussion) and AC (after concussion).

At first, we assumed that everything would be fine. The doctors all suggested "brain rest," so she rested her brain. No school. No reading. No TV. She was prepared to be bored for the two weeks that it would apparently take for her brain to get back to normal. When the two weeks were up, we made her go back to school, thinking everything would be fine. It wasn't fine, and we had no idea what was coming.

Every day by 10 a.m., I got a call from the school nurse. Her words were always the same.

"You need to come get her."

Although she would start the day in her classroom, my daughter's headaches were brutal, and she couldn't stay upright for long. The nurse provided a welcoming place to lie down, but she could only spend so much time in the nurse's office. For a few months, we played this absurd game. Every single day, I took her to school, went to work, waited anxiously for the phone call, picked her up, and tried to work from home. She tried to be brave, then fell apart, cried, screamed, and sank deeper and deeper into hopelessness. She was consumed by the ice picks that she felt in both eyes. Nothing made it better, but plenty of things made it worse. She couldn't tolerate light, sound, being upright, or moving her head. When we didn't understand the depth of her suffering, she fired verbal daggers at us and my heart broke.

Our little family was descending into a dank and frightening cave. We were all stumbling along, blind, with our hands stretched out in front of us feeling frantically for a path that would take us back into the sun. We saw this doctor, that specialist, another therapist. We bought special glasses, reading boards, melatonin, and electrostimulation units. Nothing helped and no one knew what to do. Her dad and I oscillated between being overly accommodating and trying to stick to normal routines. My older daughter was livid when her sister didn't have to do her chores "just because her head hurts."

After a while, my daughter's friends pulled away. She was cranky and couldn't do anything fun, so she became invisible. Going to school began to seem pointless. She was excused from tests, spent the whole day in the nurse's office, and felt lonelier there than at home.

I made a folder on my computer called "homeschooling."

I met with my boss and spilled my guts. The upshot was that I either had to bring my daughter to work with me every day or I had to quit. He was kind and understanding, and we christened an unused desk as her new school. After some mama bear moments, her school agreed to give her credit for the year if she completed the required assignments from home. In my fantasies, I would make lesson plans, she would do her work independently, and I would send it in to the school to be graded. Everything was going to be just fine.

In the months that she spent at school on partial brain rest, an important detail had been overlooked. My daughter could no longer read. In the BC era, she had been an excellent student in a college-prep private school. Now, she could barely and haltingly sound out the words of her textbooks to me, but she had no idea what the words meant. So much for her and I working independently, side by side.

Hard stop.

"We need a new plan," I told myself.

My eyes were suddenly wide open, and I realized that if we just kept waiting for her to get better, that might never happen. I put on my captain's hat and decided that I was now in charge of this recovery ship. This new perspective lifted the fog that had been occluding my vision. Now that I was paying attention, I saw all the ways that my

AC daughter was different from my BC daughter. I acknowledged the untreated depression and anxiety that were contributing to her suffering. I realized that she no longer swallowed normally, and sometimes she screamed because swallowed pills, or food, came out of her nose. I recognized that her personality had acutely changed, and her verbal filter was gone. I noticed that she was having trouble understanding speech, especially in a loud room. But also, she had developed a brand-new creative side that I had never seen before.

A powerful question bubbled up in me from some inner source: "I wonder what this experience will mean for her."

It would clearly mean something. Maybe it would destroy her life. Maybe she'd live in our basement forever. Maybe she'd kill herself. I thought all those options were possibilities. But I also held space for other outcomes. Maybe she'd become a healer of some sort. Maybe a neurologist. Or a psychologist. Maybe she'd develop a deep spirituality. Maybe she'd become an artist.

I started to regularly raise this query with her. "I wonder what this experience will mean for you."

I was firm that we weren't supposed to fill in the answer now. We weren't even allowed to. We just made space for the question. We let it hang there. She probably thought that I was annoying and stupid, but I believed that when the time was right the answer would appear.

It took about two years.

In that time, she had nerve injections and surgery on her neck. She did vision therapy, neurofeedback, psychotherapy, Eye Movement Desensitization and Reprocessing (EMDR), and tons of physical therapy. She had massages and craniosacral therapy, and if she hadn't refused it, she would have had acupuncture. She got hearing aids and took antidepressants. Little by little, light filtered back into her world.

We found her a school for bright kids with reading challenges, and she thrived there. She played with her pet rats and started yoga. She cut her long hair into a mohawk and asked if I would help her learn to shoot a gun. Gulp. I balked at that one, but when she explained that she was trying to reclaim her power, what could I say? Off we went to the gun range. I paid for multiple piercings, and she planned the tattoos that she would get when she was eighteen. With verbal and written language tougher than they used to be, she taught herself American Sign Language (ASL).

Out of the blue one day, she said, "I know the answer."

I had no idea what she was talking about.

"The answer. To 'what will this experience mean for me.' I know the answer," she said.

My breath caught and prickly tears crept into my eyes. Afraid of unleashing an emotional flood that would shut her up, I just waited.

She explained to me that this whole hellish experience had pushed her to tap into a deep strength and power that she had never felt before. She was certain that if she had stayed at her previous school, as the quiet and shy girl in a kitty cat T-shirt, she would never have metamorphosized into the pierced, mohawked, gun shooting, passionate photographer that she had become. She had discovered a career passion of using ASL to help kids with autism and arranged to attend a summer program at Gallaudet, a university for the deaf and hard of hearing. She found beloved friends there and, more importantly, she found a vision for her future that hadn't, after all, been permanently lost.

She had waded through a lot of poop, and she had learned to find her flowers.

Every intense experience will mean something to the people it touches. Some people facing difficult experiences become bitter and hard, some people descend into dense depression. Yet sometimes, a rough experience can spur the person facing it to find unexpected flowers. They might set new boundaries and learn to say no. They might meet a new friend or adopt a beloved pet. Sometimes, new passions emerge, or new rose gardens are planted. Your experience will mean something to you whether you want it to or not. There will likely be meanings that are positive and those that are less so. Acknowledging the negative meanings has value and it is important not to sweep them under the rug, but with flower glasses on you can often find a positive component in even the toughest experiences.

One of my patients was a woman in her fifties who was dying from breast cancer. I saw her in the hospital, and she was sad but resigned. She had three daughters who adored their mom, and they were all at the bedside in tears. There had been some conflict between the daughters that seemed to have dissolved as they all squeezed into her tiny hospital room and shared how much they loved her. The youngest daughter was particularly distraught.

She was in her late twenties and told her mom, "I can't do this without you. I just can't. I can't survive without you. You're my best friend."

As a mom of daughters, myself, this young woman's pain got to me. I blinked back tears because I didn't want to add my own emotions to this intense moment. I expected my patient, the mom, to dissolve into sobs at this raw expression of her daughter's pain. When I imagined myself in her place, I thought that's certainly what I would have done. But that's not what happened.

In a kind but no-nonsense voice, she told her daughter, "You will be fine. I've probably allowed you to become too dependent on me, and I'm sorry about that. You are strong and brave, and your sisters will help you. You will miss me, but you have your own life to live, and you will be fine."

She turned to her other daughters and said, "I know there has been some tension between you all, but it is time for that to stop. You are sisters and you need to be there for each other."

My patient didn't fall apart. She didn't even cry. Instead, she showed up for her terrified daughter as a firm but loving parent. She was a powerhouse, and I was blown away by her resolve and her bravery.

Her daughters hugged each other and cried and promised their mom that they would stick together and support each other. When I chatted with my patient later, alone, she shared how important that experience had been for her. Her daughters had been in conflict and her younger daughter seemed overly attached and was having trouble launching. My patient had been concerned about both of these dynamics and hadn't been sure what to do about them. She felt certain that something fundamental had shifted in that family meeting. She believed that her daughters would now put aside their inconsequential grievances and grow closer. She shared that she didn't think that her younger daughter, who was almost thirty, would ever detach from her sufficiently to become independent as long as she still had her mother to rely on. So, while she certainly wasn't happy to be leaving her family, she expressed that it might be better for her younger daughter in the long run.

Even in the most challenging, difficult, or sad circumstances there are flowers. The practice of looking for those flowers will change your experience of the difficult circumstance. Actually, it will change your life. I'm not saying that you will suddenly be happy about your loved one's illness or your own (my patient would certainly have given up those flowers if she could magically make her cancer disappear), but it will change your relationship to them. You don't have to look for the flowers if you don't want to, and the process will be harder for some people than for others. Yet, for every single one of us, putting on our flower glasses is worth a try. They may be dark and smudged at first and that's okay. If you keep putting them on, they will get clearer over time.

Find your flower glasses. If you aren't ready to put them on just yet, that's okay. Just lay them, metaphorically, on your nightstand so they are right there when you are ready.

Examples of finding "flowers" in difficult experiences

- Recognizing your personal strength
- Finding a new interest or passion
- Connecting with new people
- Finding deeper connections with the people in your life
- Learning to slow down
- Having a new experience
- Learning a new skill
- Reorganizing your priorities
- Letting go of toxic people
- Saying no to things you don't want to do
- Deepening your spiritual connection

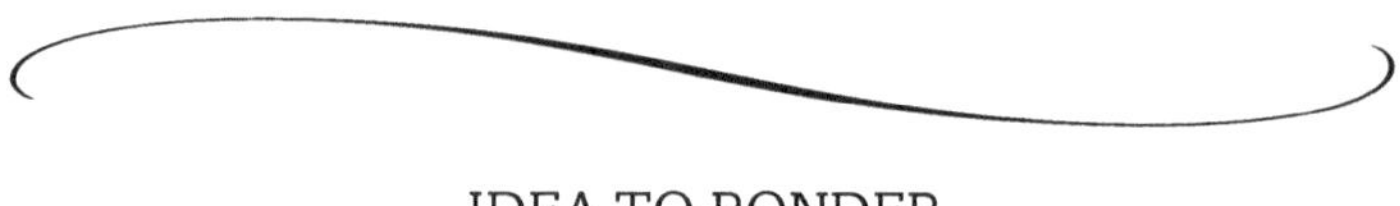

IDEA TO PONDER

In your past, when have you been able to find "flowers in the poop?"

FAMILY DISCUSSION QUESTION

If we all put on our 'flower glasses,' what flowers might we find right now?

EXERCISE

"What will this experience mean for me/you/us?"

- Write this question on a sticky note and put it up where you can see it
- Take notes on your phone or in a journal as ideas come to you
- Don't rush to answer the question, but allow the answer to emerge over time

CHAPTER 2

You Do You, Boo

"Feel this," Sherry said as she lifted up her shirt, showing me the side of her right breast.

I was visiting from out of town with my husband and two little girls, and my childhood friend Sherry had popped over to give me a hug. Her request seemed like an afterthought. She'd felt a little something odd and thought she'd ask her friend's professional opinion.

We were chatting about insignificant things as I put my hand on her breast. That moment is frozen in my memory like a still photo. I see the room we were standing in, hear the rushing in my ears, and feel the rock-hard mass.

"What do you think?" she asked with a light and lilting voice.

I had never prepared the answer to this question. What do you say when you're certain that your forty-year-old best friend has breast cancer, and you desperately don't want to be the person who tells her? The memory stops with my words frozen in my throat. I don't remember what I said. I just remember how it felt trying not to say anything.

Sherry got the official news from her doctor, and reluctantly got on the breast cancer treatment train. She did all the things they told her to do: surgery, chemotherapy, and radiation, but she didn't resonate with the uplifting, let's go pink, breast cancer experience. She toughed it out, took care of her ten-year-old daughter the best that she could, shaved her head, and puked in the bathroom. She didn't have the "I'll just work full time and take a nap when I get home" kind of cancer journey.

Others walking the road that Sherry was on found strength from wearing pink T-shirts, sporting pink ribbons, and gathering teams for breast cancer fundraising walks. But this approach didn't work for Sherry. Cancer sucked and she didn't want anyone to try to pretty it up.

She felt a pressure, from no one in particular, about how she was supposed to 'do' breast cancer. She was supposed to join groups and raise money and be positive and sit up front at survivorship events. For many people with breast cancer, this sense of community and shared purpose is vital to getting through an otherwise exhausting and wholly unpleasant ordeal. Pink Power is great if it gives you a sense of meaning and connects you with like-minded people who get you. These structures were created because they help people. Unless they don't. For Sherry, the pressure to embrace pink ribbons nagged at her like a splinter. She did crave community, however; and she ultimately found her people through the YWCA. They were all women with breast cancer, and they met regularly at a fancy hotel pool.

"None of them wore pink," Sherry told me. "All of them are mad and we talked a lot about how much we hate cancer, how to manage the sh*tty symptoms of chemo, and how our families were coping."

The important message here is 'you do you, boo.' No person's or family's illness journey is like anyone else's, and I encourage your whole family to stand up to anyone who tries to tell you how to behave or what to feel or which clubs to join. It doesn't matter what helped them or their grandma or their neighbor across the alley. There is no right way to 'do' illness, which means there is no wrong way either.

This pressure to be, or think, a certain way about managing a complex illness can originate from outside your family, but it can also come from within. Perhaps everyone in your family is always in total agreement about what each player should do, think, work on, or say. If that's true, you should probably play the lottery because you have a unicorn family with an oversized share of luck. If you have a family like the rest of us, everyone has an opinion.

"Mom shouldn't watch so much TV," one of your siblings might say.

Another might declare, "Dad needs to have a more positive attitude."

Maybe the opinion arrows come your way, "You need to cook healthier food for her," or, "You should clean the house more often."

Or maybe you shoot some of those opinion arrows yourself.

It is important to point out that many of those opinions have truth kernels within them. You or your opinion-sharing loved ones may have extremely good ideas. Healthy food and clean houses are great, and too much TV is not ideal. Yet just because an opinion has merit doesn't mean anyone else is obligated to listen to it. Should your dad who has lung cancer quit smoking? Of course. But does it help your family's coping to harp on dad's smoking once he has entered hospice? Nope. If you have a potentially helpful opinion, feel free to share it once. Maybe twice. No more than three times. Once you've shared your opinion over and over, no matter how helpful it is, the chance that your loved one will change their behavior or attitude the next time you tell them what to do is approximately zero percent. Your beautifully crafted advice will be labeled as 'nagging' in your loved one's mind, and it will go into the section of their brain labeled 'things I don't want to hear about anymore and have no intention of changing.' It won't change their behavior, but it could harm your relationship.

Sherry had a difficult breast cancer experience. Is it possible that joining fundraising groups would have helped her find meaning in her experience? Could it have helped her cope? Sure, it's possible. But what do you think it would have done to our relationship if I repeatedly sent her invitations to breast cancer walks after she had made her feelings about these things clear? She probably would have felt disrespected and angry. She would not have felt seen and supported in her unique cancer journey. My need to impose my opinion on her experience could have fractured our friendship and left her feeling lonelier than before.

Luckily, I kept my mouth shut, and twenty years later she is still one of my dearest friends.

The central idea here is that everyone's journey is their journey. And no one's journey is like anyone else's. That goes for you, your loved one who is ill, and everyone else in your family and extended community. Try to focus most of your energy on figuring out what *you* need to have or do or think to keep going on this challenging road. If you have a medical question, such whether it's okay for your father to eat so much sugar, then it makes sense to ask the doctor. But other than medical requirements, like taking medications or showing up to appointments, see if you can allow your loved one to walk their own journey, even if they are doing it differently than you think they should.

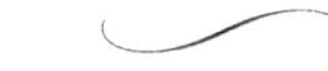

When I was in labor with my second baby, the pain got too intense when I hit eight cm and I just couldn't take it anymore. I asked for an epidural, but when the anesthesiologist got there, I told him that I just wanted a "mini-epidural."

"I don't know what that means," he said.

In between contractions that took my breath away, I told him that I wanted to feel the birth, but I just didn't want to feel it this much.

"You're telling me that you want to feel pain."

He said it like a statement, not a question.

"Yes, I guess that's what I'm saying. I want to feel the birth. Can you please just take it down a few notches?" I asked.

He couldn't let it go.

"You understand that I can take all the pain away, right?"

Of course, I understood. I was a doctor for God's sake.

"I just want a lower dose than you usually use," I squeaked out. "Can you please do that for me?"

He sighed a big sigh and said, "Well . . . I guess I can do that. No one has ever asked me for pain before. No one. Ever!"

I felt judged. Who was that guy to tell me how to give birth to my baby?

Everyone's experience and needs are different. Your job is to figure yourself out and ask for what *you*, and your loved one, want. Do you want to talk to the hospital doctor one more time because a question just occurred to you? Do you want to leave your loved one's bedside and go home to take a shower? Do you want to hire some caregiving help so you can get a break? There is no need for excuses, explanations, guilt, or self-doubt. You want what you want and that's just fine. That goes for your loved ones, too.

Debbie shouted the news of her ovarian cancer from the rooftops. All her social media friends knew her cancer stage, her drug names, and when she lost her hair. She used her hatred of the whole cancer nightmare to fuel her through the tough times, and she got strength from the caring community that circled around her. She proudly shared her bald or scarf-adorned head and didn't bother to buy a wig.

Francis took a different approach.

She told only her closest family members and a couple of friends about her advanced pancreatic cancer. She turned down social invitations and gracefully bowed out of family events. Her sister took her to buy a wig even before her hair fell out and she wore it every time she left the house. No one suspected the hell that she was going through, and most people in her world didn't even know that she had cancer until she died.

You probably have an opinion about which approach is 'better.' I think I know what I will do if I ever find myself in this situation. But if Debbie or Francis were your loved one, their approach is none of your business. If the urge bubbles up to tell Debbie that she should be a little more discrete or to tell Francis that she shouldn't be so secretive, do your best to prevent those words from leaving your mouth.

Full disclosure, I am personally in Debbie's camp. When my time comes to have a thing that threatens my life, you will probably all know about it. I am stressed out by secrets and feel lighter when I share. Early in my career I, mistakenly, assumed that this was the right approach for everyone. I used to encourage my private-leaning patients to share their struggle widely so that people could gather around them and lift them up. I was certain that this way was the "better" way, and I tried to help them get over their resistance to sharing. If you were my patient back then, please accept my apology. It was arrogant and narcissistic of me to assume that my way is *the* way. There are many ways to cope, and our general approach should be to help our loved ones figure out *their* way and then help them to manifest it.

There is one caveat to keep in mind. Some people isolate because they are depressed, and this does not support their well-being. We'll dive deeper into this in a later chapter, but for now let's assume that your loved one wants privacy because they want privacy, not because they're depressed.

The other thing to tease out here is shame. It is insane that people facing serious illness feel shame about being sick, but sometimes shame sneaks into the most unwelcome places. The shame may show up when the illness impacts a certain part of the body, like the genitals or gastrointestinal tract, or sometimes when an illness is associated, irrelevantly and often incorrectly, with a lifestyle choice, such as lung cancer or AIDS. Sometimes it shows up when a cancer is somewhat unusual, like breast cancer in a man. Sometimes people bring their own shame down generations; if all the men in a family got diabetic kidney disease when they got "old," a younger man's self-concept might be threatened if his kidneys start to fail. Sometimes the shame comes when a body looks different after treatment.

If a breast or leg is gone, or speech is no longer fluid after a stroke, shame may whisper, "you aren't valuable anymore."

Let's pitch illness shaming straight out the window. Your loved one, and you, are valuable because of your insides, not your outsides. The Universe doesn't care how many legs you have or whether your breasts look different than they used to.

It is important to realize that your loved one's moodiness or sadness may have a touch of shame attached. While you can't return their body to how it used to be, you *can* share your affection and reverence for their sweet soul, loving heart, or hilarious sense of humor.

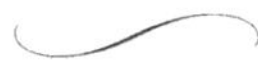

PLEASE READ THIS TO THE PERSON WITH THE ILLNESS

A note for the person facing illness:

Just like no doctor or friend or loved one should be allowed to impose their will upon you, telling you how to behave or how to feel or how to "do" your illness, shame should not be given a shame gun and allowed to spew its nasty goo all over you. Illness stinks and it isn't your fault. Even if you secretly feel like it's your fault because you drank a case of beer every day or had sex without condoms or ate a lot of chocolate chip cookies, it still isn't your fault. There are plenty of drunk cookie eaters having unprotected sex who aren't facing illness right now. No one knows why some people get a serious illness and others don't.

It isn't your fault.

It isn't your fault.

It isn't your fault.

And if anyone in your life has the gall to imply that it's even a little bit your fault, they're wrong. It isn't your fault.

There is nothing shameful about having an illness, no matter where it is on your body or how it has changed you. That shame voice in your head is a nasty liar and I want you to start talking back to it.

If a mean voice in your head says, "You can't go out looking like that," stand up tall, throw your shoulders back, jut out your chin, lift your eyebrows and say, "EXCUSE ME?!?!" with all the attitude you can muster.

Choose a comeback and practice it until it sits on the tip of your tongue.

"I am a child of the Universe/God/My Mama, and I am beautiful/perfect/just fine/enough just as I am."

You'll probably have to say it over and over and over, but that's okay. Every time you say it, your shame shrinks a little and your self-acceptance grows.

If you are feeling depressed, I want you to tell your doctor because depression is treatable, and you deserve to feel better. Once you're certain that depression and shame aren't clouding your view, I want you to plant your flag firmly in the "this is how I want to do it" ground.

This is your illness, and you get to "do" your illness any way you want to.

Back to you, dear caregiver.

The one who is showing up, caring, supporting, doing laundry, filling pill boxes, and serving as an unpaid Uber driver. This is your journey, too.

As the caregiver, you get to help in the way that works for you. You could do a lot or a little. You could do it all yourself or hire people to do some of the tasks that you don't enjoy. You can take time off work or work full time. Here's what you shouldn't do: give and give and give until you are holding on by the tips of your fingernails and about to crash to the ground.

Please don't do this.

We all, flawed humans that we are, seem to spend an inordinate amount of energy criticizing ourselves and each other. We beat ourselves up for being cranky, tired, and imperfect, and we try to manipulate each other's behavior so that we feel safe and in control. Let's all agree not to participate in that craziness. Caring for someone with a serious illness can be brutal, so you deserve to be treated with kindness—especially from yourself. And when has telling someone else how to be or what to think ever worked? It just creates resentment and hard feelings, and who wants that when your family is doing their best to stay afloat in stormy weather?

Try to check in with yourself and figure out what you need. Then, lovingly and non-judgmentally communicate that to your people. When necessary, look for compromises. You want to tell everyone about your mom's cancer, and she wants to keep it quiet? Ask her if you can tell your three closest friends if they promise not to tell anyone else. Then write about the whole experience in your private journal, so you can unload the tough stuff without compromising your mom's need for privacy. You want your dad to take a bunch of dietary supplements, but he doesn't want to? Ask his doctor for assurance that they aren't dangerous, try once or twice to explain to him why you think they would be helpful, and then respect your dad's "no" if it persists.

I know this isn't easy.

When facing a serious illness, in yourself or someone you love, attempts at control often feel safer than letting go. Unfortunately, they usually don't work. People resist being controlled and trying to impose your point of view on someone else creates friction. During rough times, it works better when everyone sticks together. Imagine standing side by side, arm in arm, helping each other resist the storm. Will your loved one make decisions that you vehemently disagree with? Definitely. Should they listen to you? Probably, but they also have every right to follow their own internal compass and ignore all your great advice. If you attempt to overrule their point of view it can fracture your connection just when family connection is most crucial.

If you feel the urge to tell your frustrating loved one, who never listens to you, for the tenth time why your way is the best way, take three slow, deep breaths and gently ask yourself the following question:

Would I rather be right, or would I rather be happy?

I'll bet that some of the advice that you share with your loved one is excellent. It might even be brilliant. You have agonized over their well-being, searched far corners of the internet for sage advice, and talked to friends, colleagues, doctors, and healers of all kinds. You just want to help and share what you've learned. Things would be better if only your loved one would listen to you.

I get it.

Even without knowing you, I agree with you. Family members often have great ideas, and if you picked up this book you are clearly a seeker who is looking for ways to make things better. But here's the problem: if your loved one is over eighteen with an intact ability to make their own decisions, their questionable choices are none of your business.

I can hear your "Yes, but . . ." bubbling up.

"You don't understand," you might say.

She has decided to stop treatment or become a Wiccan or get coffee enemas. I hear you. This is not how you would conduct yourself and you do not approve.

You make good points. You want him to come live with you or walk more or drink kombucha. You have all the reasons and the evidence, but he still won't listen to you. It can be exasperating.

Each piece of unfollowed advice can feel like it is life or death. You may feel like it is your duty to make your loved one eat more or eat less, get out of bed or go back to bed, take a dietary supplement or leave the cookies in the cabinet.

"How can she get better if she doesn't eat?!" you might ask in frustration.

Again, if your loved one can understand the consequences of their actions, *they* are responsible for their decisions. Full stop. You know who is not responsible for making a cognitively intact sentient being over the age of eighteen do something that they don't want to do? You.

People that you love can be frustrating. They don't always appreciate your research or wise ideas, and they may even get annoyed with you when you are just trying to help.

"Just back off," your sister or brother or mom or dad might say.

This can be hard to hear.

Backing off is tough

When life is stressful, *doing* can feel easier than *being*. When you stop buzzing around, sad or scary feelings can seep in, and you may be subconsciously working hard to keep them out. However, even if *doing* feels easier than *being*, it is not always the best approach. You might feel compelled to dive into an exhaustive internet search about your brother's condition, purge the frayed towels from your mom's linen closet or buy a top-of-the-line recliner to heave your dad to a stand when it's time for dinner. If they would only understand how helpful you can be, things would be better, right? Yet your dad might hate recliners and your mom might love her ratty towels.

If your loved one is facing a serious illness, spending high-quality time just *being* with them is vitally important. See if you can spend some time with your person without making any suggestions. None. Don't tell them what they should eat or how much, don't show them print outs from the internet of overseas treatments and don't clean their messy house without asking first. If that seems impossible, make your great suggestions a couple of times, then if your loved one doesn't go for it, do your very best to simply let it go. At a time when family connection is crucially important, remember to ask yourself the question:

Would I rather be right, or would I rather be happy?

See if you can refocus your efforts from trying to influence each other's behavior to, instead, trying to help each other cope.

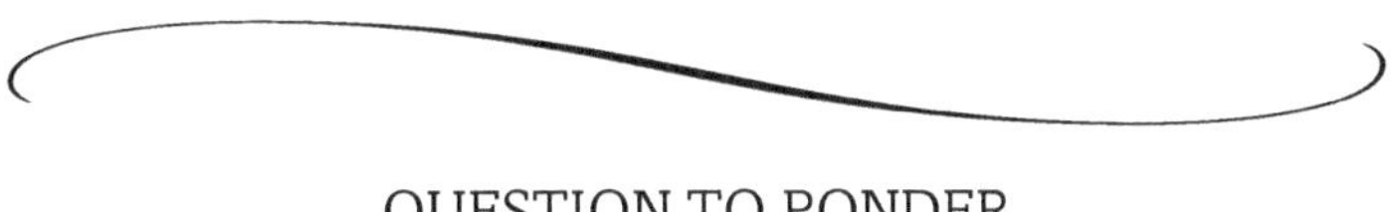

QUESTION TO PONDER

Is your family generally supportive of each other's quirkiness and individuality, or is there a pressure for everyone in the family to see things the same way?

FAMILY DISCUSSION QUESTION

What does each person in the family need to feel supported in their individual style of coping?

EXERCISE

Have everyone in the family answer these questions:

"The things that I do to help me cope are______."
"Three things that others could do to help me cope are________."

After committing to not judging or getting defensive, share your answers with each other.

CHAPTER 3

Manage the Medical Machine

When Francis was in his late eighties he fell. He was a robust and intellectual man, married to his high school sweetheart. He read the *New York Times* cover to cover every day and did the crossword puzzle on Sundays. Francis was the keystone of his close-knit family and none of them had ever imagined a world without his robust and commanding presence. Then a loose throw rug upended his future and enrolled his family in a crash course on managing the medical machine.

"My husband fell. I can't get him up," Francis's wife told the 911 operator in a shaky voice.

"Don't worry, Ma'am. We'll send someone to help him out," the operator reassured her.

The paramedics came quickly. They were kind and efficient, and within a few minutes Francis was strapped onto a stretcher on his way to the hospital. That's when it all got crazy.

The emergency room was packed, and Francis spent hours on a stretcher in the hallway while the emergency department physicians and nurses worked to save patients facing heart attacks, strokes, and motor vehicle accidents. Family members weren't allowed in the emergency department because of the COVID-19 pandemic, so Francis had no supportive person to help him pass the time or reassure him that he would be okay. His hearing aids were back at home on his bedside table, and he was exhausted, frightened, and in pain. After a while he exploded.

"Can someone help me?!?" he yelled out. "HELLO! CAN SOMEBODY HELP ME?!?"

A resident checked on him briefly and gave instructions to the nurse. Soon she had started an intravenous line and pushed two mystery medicines into his blood stream. He felt fuzzy-headed and sleepy.

When he woke up a few hours later, Francis was different.

As he was wheeled to his hospital room, Francis mumbled to himself and picked at his blankets. He didn't recognize that man who was pushing his bed and he couldn't have told you where he was going. The transporter saw him as a confused, elderly man and spoke to him in a distracted tone.

"I'm taking you to your room now, okay?"

Francis didn't answer.

The admitting physician called Francis's wife, Vicky, to update her on his condition.

"His right hip is broken," the doctor said matter-of-factly. "The orthopedic surgeon will be by in the morning to see him."

"Is he going to be okay?" Vicky asked with a quivering voice. "Can I come see him?"

"Sure, you can come see him," the doctor told her. "Hip fracture is serious in an older person. We'll have to see how it goes. We'll manage his pain and see what ortho says tomorrow."

Vicky felt the heaviness of a hundred unanswered questions, but she couldn't formulate any of them clearly enough to ask them out loud.

She rushed to the hospital to see her husband, but the man she found in Francis's bed didn't seem like her husband at all. Francis called her Brenda, his first wife's name, and she couldn't stop him from yelling.

"CAN SOMEBODY HELP ME?!?!" he called out with a booming voice. "Help me, help me, help me, help me, HELP ME!"

"I'm right here," Vicky said, over and over, but Francis wouldn't calm down. Vicky was mortified, and she was terrified.

She called his nurse and asked her to check on Francis. The nurse came to his bedside, patted his hand, and said "Now Mr. Francis, you need to calm down. You're getting everybody all upset."

"He'll be OK," she told Vicky. "You should get some rest."

The next morning, Francis seemed a bit more like himself. He recognized Vicky and asked for a cup of coffee. A young man, who looked like a college student, showed up wearing a short white coat and started asking Francis ridiculous questions.

"Who is the president?" he asked. "What is today's date?"

Vicky found these questions insulting. Francis read the paper every day and was the smartest man she knew. This "doctor" was treating him like he was stupid, and she was getting increasingly annoyed.

When Francis got every question except his name wrong, Vicky started to cry.

"What is wrong with him?" Vicky asked the young man in the white coat. "This isn't him. I don't understand what is happening."

"Well, he clearly has dementia," the young man said in an authoritative tone.

"Dementia?" Vicky repeated with a question in her voice. "No one ever told us he has dementia." She asked nervously, "Did he hit his head or something?"

"No," the man said. "We did a CT of his head and it's fine."

The young man left without any further explanation and Vicky spent hours at Francis's bedside trying to hold herself together. What did he mean when he said that Francis was 'fine?' Francis either slept or screamed "ouch!" or "help," and he kicked at the nurses when they tried to take care of him. He was the polar opposite of fine.

Every few hours a nurse would put medicine in his intravenous line and usually after that, he slept.

Another young doctor came in and asked her if they should "pound on his chest" and "put a tube in his throat" if he needed it.

"Of course!" Vicky said.

A third young doctor burst into the room, talking at double speed.

"Hi! I'm from orthopedics. We can fix up Mr. Francis's hip but there are risks, including infection and even death. I hope he'll regain the ability to walk, but I can't guarantee it. Even if everything turns out fine, he won't be able to go home right after surgery, he'll need to go to rehab for a few weeks. I want you to talk to the palliative care team before you make the decision about surgery. They should be by soon. If you decide to go ahead with surgery, I'll be back later." The door closed behind the doctor before Vicky could even think of a question to ask.

Palliative care? Did that mean he was dying? Would fixing his hip save his life? But the doctor said he could die from the surgery. The air in Francis's room felt heavy and oppressive and Vicky couldn't sit still. She felt like her world was collapsing. She didn't know what had happened to her beloved husband, and all she could think about was that she had lost the man she'd spent her life with. He might never be the same, and he might die. Vicky couldn't fathom life without Francis, and she felt completely overwhelmed, terrified, and powerless. She sat by his bedside, held his hand, and cried.

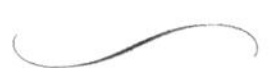

What happened here?

Francis was doing well, broke his hip, went to the hospital, and then fell apart. Multiple doctors of unclear experience levels communicated with Francis's wife about scary topics that left her worried and confused. Now Francis wasn't doing well, and his wife wasn't doing well either.

The Medical Machine Explained

When an older person breaks a hip, the risk of permanent decline in function is substantial. Some patients recover completely, while others are never quite the same. For some people, surgical repair of a broken hip is the obvious choice, while for others (particularly those with long-standing, severe dementia), medical management is a reasonable alternative. Palliative care clinicians can help families understand what is going on and help them make decisions that take into account both the medical reality and the family's goals.

Because many people, including physicians, don't understand exactly what palliative care clinicians do, they may not be called in to help even when a palliative care consult would be of great benefit to the family. Palliative care teams help with symptom management, coping, and medical decisions, and are appropriate for anyone with a serious illness, including an older person with a hip fracture. The common misconception that palliative care is just for dying people is completely inaccurate. Francis's medical team did the right thing by consulting palliative care, but because they didn't explain their reasoning to Vicky, she was left with the (inaccurate) assumption that this meant that Francis was going to die.

In an older person, who may have mild unrecognized cognitive deficits, going to the hospital can precipitate an acute, and often temporary, decline in cognitive function. The confusion may be related to pain, medications, and a condition called 'sundowning' that causes older people to become confused at night and more oriented during the day.

Francis likely received medication for pain, and possibly anxiety, when he started yelling in the emergency department. This may have been the precipitating factor that resulted in his agitated confusion and his wife's terrified tears.

One of the multiple white coat-clad people who spoke to Francis's wife stated definitively, after meeting him once, that Francis has dementia.

"Dementia?! No." his wife thought. "No. I can't possibly handle that."

The statement that Francis has dementia sent Vicky down a dark spiral staircase of terror as she remembered the suffering of her friend, whose husband had spent a decade withering away from dementia.

The problem is the definitive statement that Francis had dementia was wrong.

Dementia is generally a slowly progressive disease, so a man like Francis who was doing the *New York Times* crossword puzzle last week does not have dementia this week. However, what he might have had is delirium. These two conditions can mimic each other, and they are sometimes confused.

While dementia doesn't appear suddenly after twenty-four hours in the hospital, delirium commonly does just that. Delirium is a state of confusion or disorientation that usually starts suddenly, and it can be brought on by medications, sleep deprivation, hospitalization, pain, surgery, and other disruptions to the person's regular routine. It can be both hypoactive (the person is sleepy and slow to respond) or hyperactive (the person is agitated and restless). Francis had hyperactive delirium.

If it is so clear that Francis had agitated delirium, why did the young "doctor" say it was dementia? That happened because the doctor wasn't actually a doctor quite yet. He was learning to be a doctor, and he simply made a mistake. While it was not his intention, he dramatically increased Francis's wife's suffering. His casual words had a power over her wellbeing that he had not yet learned to wield with precision and compassion. He probably didn't even remember this small nugget of communication, but Francis's wife will never forget it.

Many people came into Francis's room that day; how was his wife supposed to know who to listen to and which information to believe?

Student doctors, also called medical students, practice caring for patients as part of their schooling. They can't write prescriptions or medical orders, but they *are* assigned patients and sent into rooms to examine patients and talk to families. They can often offer great comfort to families because they have more time to spend in each room, but they can also inadvertently cause distress if they say something that isn't quite right.

While it isn't universally true, in many hospitals medical students wear short white coats while residents and senior doctors (called attendings) wear longer coats that come to the knee. If a "doctor" in a short white coat tells you something that doesn't seem quite right, be sure to confirm it with a longer coat doctor. You might even want to confirm one more time with a longer coat doctor who has a few wrinkles or grey hairs.

Before he broke his hip, Francis had strong cognitive skills and his wife was shocked at his sudden and severe decline after admission to the hospital. She couldn't understand how breaking his hip could so profoundly change his personality, and because she was overwhelmed, she couldn't even formulate clear questions to ask the doctor. She felt panicked, confused, and paralyzed.

Managing the Medical Machine

Could anything have been done to make this experience less traumatic for Francis's wife?

While it would have been nice if one kind and experienced doctor could have spent an hour chatting with Vicky, reassuring and supporting her, the current medical climate makes that ideal unlikely. Physicians and nurses are caring for more patients than they have in the past, and their administrative burdens have skyrocketed. They are overwhelmed and exhausted and generally doing their best. Yet their best isn't perfect, so it is a good idea to have a self-advocacy plan that you can whip out whenever you need to interact with the medical machine.

Advocacy 101

1. Create a Strong Team
2. Emphasize Your Loved One's Baseline Function
3. Consider The Source of Information
4. Confirm Key Information
5. Be on Alert
6. Write Down Your Questions
7. Take Notes
8. Organize the Information
9. Have a Prevention Point of View
10. Fill Up Your Own Cup

1. Create a Strong Team

Your advocacy team can include family, friends, acquaintances, and anyone else who cares about you and is willing to help. It is a good idea to create a diverse advocacy team, because coping with a serious illness takes a village. Team members may include (but are not limited to) a spouse or partner, siblings, children, friends, neighbors, work colleagues, people in your faith community, knitting partners, people in your running club, and fellow tiny dog enthusiasts. Try to think outside the box. Who else in your world might be able to help in some way? These people can accompany your loved one to doctor visits, bake vegetarian lasagna, rake the leaves, bring over fancy chocolates, commiserate when a favorite sports team loses, or show up for late night conversations about life and death.

Many hospitals prefer that a family choose one spokesperson to communicate with the medical team, so the doctors don't need to say the same thing over and over to each of your twenty-three cousins. The spokesperson can then communicate with the rest of the advocacy team. If your loved one is able to share their opinion, they can help choose the family spokesperson. If not, gather the key people and choose a person with strong communication skills. The family spokesperson may be the medical power of attorney, or they may not. More on that in chapter four.

Your advocacy team can also help you create a strong *medical* team.

Creating a strong medical team is crucial for getting the best possible medical care. Every person's team will be different, so a personalized approach is ideal. Most people won't need all these practitioners, but your loved one will probably need at least a few. Look over the list and see if adding one or two of these experts to your loved one's team might be helpful.

- Primary care physician to manage their outpatient care—everyone should have this

- Geriatrician for expertise in caring for older people

- Hospitalist to manage their hospital-based care

- Medical specialist for diagnosed conditions such as cancer, heart disease, and kidney disease

- Second opinion medical specialist for certain conditions, such as unusual cancers

- Palliative care physician if diagnosed with a serious illness, even if pursuing treatment to prolong life

- General surgeon for conditions such as gallbladder disease or appendicitis

- Surgical subspecialist for conditions such as pelvic cancers or brain tumors

- Psychotherapist or counselor to help learn coping techniques and manage stress, anxiety, depression, and trauma

- Psychiatrist to help manage complex mental health conditions

- Neuropsychologist for patients with early dementia or neurologic conditions

- Medical social worker (usually hospital-based) for help identifying resources

- Acupuncturist to help with stress, depression, anxiety, sleep, pain, symptoms of disease, and side effects of treatment, such as chemotherapy

- Manual medicine practitioner, such as a massage therapist, osteopathic physician, or chiropractor, to help with musculoskeletal pain and dysfunction

- Mind-body specialist to help learn effective relaxation techniques

- Physical therapist to help recover physical function and mobility after injury or prolonged deconditioning

- Occupational therapist to help recover function after injury or stroke

- Speech and language pathologist to help with safe swallowing and communication in people with dementia, neurologic trauma, or stroke

- Chaplain for spiritual concerns

- Home health aide to help care for your loved one at home

If you'd like some help figuring out how to put together a great medical team, you can find a helpful guide on my website: www.CopingSupport.com.

2. Emphasize Your Loved One's Baseline Function

Francis's baseline function, how he was doing before he fell, was a key piece of information that his doctors needed to know. Before he fell, he had no problem getting around and his mind was sharp. This makes it clear that he did not have dementia. It also makes it more obvious that surgical repair of his broken hip was likely the best approach. When physicians only see your loved one in their hospital bed, confused and calling out, they have no way of knowing that just last week you were debating politics or competently managing the family finances together. The visual image of a confused, frail appearing, elderly patient is so powerful that you may have to work hard to make the physician understand that your loved one was fully functional a few days before. And if that isn't the case, and your loved one has been declining for some time, that is important information for the doctor to know, as well. Treatment decisions may be different depending on how your loved one was doing before they landed in the hospital. Be sure to paint a clear picture for every doctor that you see.

Your communication with the doctors might sound something like this:

- "I think it's important that you realize that just last week Francis was doing the *New York Times* Sunday crossword puzzle all by himself. And he finished it! He didn't get confused until *after* he got to the hospital."

- "Mom has been getting a little more confused over the past six months, but she was still able to do her own grocery shopping until last Tuesday. Then she suddenly got much more confused and couldn't figure out the microwave. This was a big change in her function."

- "Dad was living alone, caring for himself, cooking dinner every night, and playing cards with friends until last week. Last week he started a new medicine and he's been dizzy, confused, and falling since then."

The more specific you can be about what your loved one used to be able to do, and when things changed, the better care the doctors will be able to provide. You'll get good at your speech because if you tell it to one doctor, you've told it to one doctor. Don't assume the information has accurately gotten passed around. Every time a new doctor or other healthcare provider comes in the room, fire that speech back up.

I learned this lesson myself when one of my long-term patients, Geoffrey, landed in the intensive care unit, bleeding from his stomach. Geoffrey had an advanced cancer, but he'd been doing well overall. During our office visit the week before his ulcer started bleeding, he'd been alert, completely oriented, and as funny as usual. But when I saw him in the ICU, he was mumbling, picking at his blankets, and he didn't acknowledge me when I called his name and took his hand. It shocked me to see how immediately his care team assumed that this was Geoffrey's baseline state. It impacted how they talked about him, how they interacted with him, and the treatment decisions that they discussed. I found myself repeating over and over, in person and in his medical record, that last week Geoffrey had been different.

I am certain that I've made that mistake myself in the past. Thanks to Geoffrey, I will never make it again.

3. Consider the Source of Information

Hospital rooms can feel like train stations. There is a constant influx of people focused on completing their assigned task and communicating in a language that you may not totally understand.

It is important to assess any information based on who is providing it. To do that you need to know who the players are.

The Hospital Players

Attending: A senior doctor who has completed residency.

Resident: A junior doctor who has graduated medical school but is still in training.

Intern: A first year resident.

Fellow: A doctor who has completed residency but is getting further specialized training, so they are not yet an attending.

Hospitalist: A doctor whose whole job is to care for hospitalized patients. They often work for a week and then get a week off, so your loved one may have several hospitalists during a long hospital stay. The hospitalist is usually the "captain of the ship" for hospitalized patients.

Medical Student: A student who is in medical school, learning to be a doctor.

Emergency Medicine Physician: The physician that will see your loved one in the emergency department, run tests, and treat emergent problems. If they think admission to the hospital is required, they will call the hospitalist or admitting physician. Insider tip: Although you might be used to referring to the place in a hospital that provides emergency care as the "ER" (an abbreviation of emergency room), people in the medical community refer to it as the "ED" (short for emergency department).

Admitting Physician: The doctor who is responsible for deciding if your loved one needs to be admitted to the hospital and for writing the admission orders. This may or may not be the same doctor who will care for the patient once they are admitted to their hospital room.

On-Call Physician: The physician who is covering the service overnight or on a weekend or holiday. This will probably not be the same person who cares for the patient in the daytime, although it could be.

Specialist: A physician with special training in a particular field such as cardiology, neurology, surgery, palliative care, etc. In some hospitals the specialists give recommendations to the hospitalist but don't write orders themselves, and in other hospitals the specialists write orders that are related to their specialty.

Nurse Practitioner: An NP is a nurse who has pursued further training (at the master's degree level) to allow them to prescribe medications and create treatment plans. Some nurses pursue a Doctorate of Nursing Practice (DNP) which allows them to use the title "doctor" in the same way that a person with a PhD uses the title doctor. They provide a valuable contribution to the healthcare team but are not physicians. Some states require that nurse practitioners are supervised by a physician, while other states allow independent practice.

Physician Assistant (or Associate): PAs are licensed healthcare professionals who pursue master's degree level training in clinical care. They are trained in the medical, rather than nursing, model. They work alongside physicians but do not, currently, practice independently. PAs are not nurses or physicians.

4. Confirm Key Information

Consider any information that you receive in light of the expertise of the person who is sharing it with you, and then confirm it with the most appropriate person. If the emergency department intern says that your loved one probably won't walk again, ask the surgeon and physical therapist what they think. If the occupational therapist says that a medication isn't right for your loved one, seek the hospitalist's opinion. If a medical student says your previously well loved one has dementia, be sure to check that out with an attending.

5. Be on Alert

Hospitals are chaotic places and, unfortunately, many thousands of people die every year from inadvertent medical errors. Physicians and nurses do their best to avoid making mistakes, but the sheer number of patients, tests, treatments, medications, and complex decisions makes errors almost inevitable. Your vigilance can prevent a medical mistake.

Perhaps the most important thing that you can do is pay attention.

"What is that blue pill?" you might ask the nurse. "She didn't have a blue pill before."

If you don't recognize the name of the medicine or know why your loved one is taking it, ask the nurse to call the doctor to confirm what it is for and that it was prescribed for the right person. If you hear a heavy sigh or get an annoyed vibe from the nurse, don't worry about it. They have the right to be annoyed, and you have the right to keep your loved one safe. You can send a basket of treats to the nurse's station at the end of the hospitalization as a thank you for putting up with you!

6. Write Down Your Questions

You may have noticed that questions come to you freely when the doctor isn't in the room and then immediately leave your mind as soon as the doctor walks in. Keep a notebook with you and jot down your questions as they come to you. When the doctor shows up, whip out your notebook and get your questions answered. If you don't understand the answer, ask again. Ask until you understand.

Asking your questions early in the visit is helpful for you and for your doctor because it helps them prioritize your concerns even when time is short.

Doctors don't like 'door handle questions.' These questions start with "Oh, just one more thing, doc," and happen after the visit is completed and the doctor has her hand on the door handle about to move on to the next patient. These questions are often the ones that the patient or family has been gathering the nerve to bring up, so they aren't usually quick and easy questions. For example, "Oh, just one more thing, doc. I haven't been able to have an erection for the last year," or, "Can you tell dad it isn't safe for him to drive anymore?"

If the doctor has mentally moved on to the next patient before you blurt out your door handle question, he might not give as much thought and attention to the question as it deserves. In the ideal world, your doctor would spend as much time with you as you want them to, but the medical Universe is not always ideal. So, if you want to get the best from your doctor, it pays to understand them. Ask your important questions up front so you aren't the door handle person.

7. Take Notes

No matter how certain you are that you will remember everything the doctor said, take notes during (or immediately after) the visit. It is shocking what leaks out of our minds a few hours after an important medical consultation has been completed. You want notes so you can remember the conversation later, but also so you can answer the inevitable question, "What did the doctor say?"

8. Organize the Information

Keep an organized notebook so you have a repository for important medical information. You can record how things are going at home, how symptoms are progressing, medical history, notes from medical consultations, and more. See below for a suggested approach to setting up your notebook. Bring the notebook to every medical encounter and make copies of important documents that you'd like the doctor to put in your loved one's medical record.

A note about symptom tracking:
Tracking your loved one's symptoms can be a great idea or a terrible one.

Sometimes, following the severity of pain and tracking how much medication is needed can help to inform treatment. Other times it can focus undue attention on the pain and make it worse. Following your loved one's bowel movements is helpful to be sure they don't go nine days without one, but if you spend too much time each day obsessing about bowel movements, everyone's quality of life will go down the toilet.

Some people find it helpful to track *positive* metrics. For example, you can track a "comfort score" rather than a pain score, or track "energy" rather than fatigue. Rather than asking your loved one "How's your pain today?" you could ask "How's your comfort today?"

Your Medical Notebook

I suggest a looseleaf notebook so you can add papers to each section as needed. Be sure you get a hole punch that matches your notebook.

Sections to Consider:
- Current medication and supplement list
- List of diagnosed medical conditions—past and current (e.g., high blood pressure, diabetes, breast cancer treated successfully with chemo/radiation). Include the year of diagnosis if you know it
- List of surgeries
- Family history if it is relevant (e.g., four people died before age fifty of heart attacks)
- Questions that you want to ask the doctor
- Medical consultations/conversations with doctors (including second opinions)
- Medication tracker (e.g., for pain or constipation medications)
- Symptom tracker (e.g., pain/comfort, nausea, bowel movements)
- Pictures if relevant (e.g., pictures of a wound over time)
- Important papers (e.g., advance directive, guardianship)
- Discharge summaries after hospitalizations (request a copy of this a few weeks after every hospital discharge)

9. Have A Prevention Point of View

Having a prevention point of view means taking steps *before* something bad happens to prevent a problem. This is the idea behind baby proofing the house when you live with a toddler; you wouldn't wait for him to drink bleach before installing cabinet locks. If you live with an older person or someone who is unsteady on their feet, be proactive about preventing falls. You can install grab bars in the shower, bath, and near the toilet. You can get rid of all the throw rugs that are terrible tripping hazards. You can move electrical cords so no one gets a foot caught in one and tumbles to the ground. If your loved one is experiencing significant cognitive decline, you can take the knobs off the stove and replace the real car keys with fake ones.

Here are some other ideas to help your loved one stay safe and get the best medical care:

- If your loved one is having a body part surgically removed or altered, write "NO!" in big letters with a black permanent marker on the wrong side of the body.

- Send your loved one's hearing aids with them to the hospital so they can communicate effectively with the medical team.

- Decorate your loved one's hospital room with things from home (if allowed) to help remind them of the people in their life.

- Leave your name and cell phone number in your loved one's hospital room so it is easy for people to contact you.

- Tell the hospital doctors if your loved one is likely to withdraw from alcohol or other substances, like cigarettes or illicit drugs, so they can be on the lookout and treat withdrawal symptoms if needed.

- Get a pill box to help your loved one manage their medications at home.

- Keep an accurate and updated list of medications and supplements. Don't forget to redo it every time a medication is added, discontinued, or there is a change in dose.

- If you hire home health aides, have a communication notebook and ask them to write in it each day. They can record events, moods, bowel movements, food intake, concerns, etc.

- If you are having trouble talking to your loved one about difficult topics, like safety at home or behind the wheel, ask a geriatrician, primary care doctor, or neuropsychologist to do it for you.

- If you have concerns that your loved one has dementia, have them formally evaluated with objective testing so you have a baseline to compare to later.

- Keep a record of medication changes and any changes in behavior so you can alert the doctors to possible medication side effects. Did Francis receive opioid pain medications or sedatives before he became delirious? Was he continuing to receive them? Maybe a medication change or dose adjustment might have helped improve his confusion. The conversation with the doctor could have gone something like this: "I notice that whenever Francis gets the pain pill and sedative, he seems to get more confused. Could we try a lower dose or different medicine?"

10. Fill Your Own Cup

Let's speak the truth: this is hard.

Caring for someone who is ill is one of the hardest things that you will ever have to do. It is fraught with fear, exhaustion, sadness, overwhelm, guilt, and if you are a human being you have felt "I am over this and I don't want to do it anymore." So, if you feel wrung out like an old wet sponge, you are totally normal.

Here's the thing . . . You can't pour from an empty cup. You can't drive with an empty gas tank. You can't shoot a gun with no bullets. Pick your favorite metaphor and then get busy filling yourself up, because you're no good to anyone if you are empty, depleted, or sick.

We'll talk more about how to fill up your cup in a later chapter, but you might as well start thinking about it now, because the biggest impediment to having a full cup is *you*.

I know, I know, I know. You're too busy. You don't have enough money or time. No one else in the family is helping so you have to do it all and there's no space left to take care of yourself. You have kids who do sports or theater, and you feel like an Uber driver. Your dog has a collapsing trachea and needs a pile of medicines three times a day. Life is a lot, and it is hard to find time for yourself. I get it.

You need to do it anyway.

If your gas gauge is on empty and you have to drive thirty minutes to get to a meeting, what do you have to do *even if you are running late?* You must stop for gas. Will it make you late to the meeting? Yes. But you know what would make you even later? Having a car that slows down against your will and coasts to the side of the road with a completely empty gas tank.

A significant portion of this book is dedicated to helping you fill up your tank.

By the end of the book, you will have a bigger toolbox to manage your own stress and fill yourself up so that life feels lighter, even as you deal with the challenges of helping a loved one with a serious illness. Filling your tank won't take away your sadness or concern for your loved one, but it will give you the energy and skills to bring your best self to the challenge.

Taking care of yourself won't make the mountain smaller, but it will buff you up so you have the strength to make the climb.

QUESTION TO PONDER

Is my gas tank full, half empty, or bone dry?

FAMILY DISCUSSION QUESTION

Do you have the right medical team in place?

EXERCISE

Make a medical tracking notebook with sections
that fit the needs of your family.

CHAPTER 4

Act in Advance

Thomas was a cheerful man in his late sixties with flyaway white hair and a warm smile that made it seem like we were old friends. When we met, Thomas was propped up in his hospital bed reading a newspaper and chatting with a quieter man who introduced himself as Jeremy.

"Hi Doc!" Thomas said brightly. "Jeremy and I are just hanging out. Want to join us?"

They had managed to create a lazy Saturday morning vibe despite the antiseptic smells and vomit basins on the windowsill.

I came to meet Thomas that day because his oncologist had requested a palliative care consult. Thomas's prostate cancer had spread despite hormones, immunotherapy, radiation, and prayer. Despite his jolly demeanor, Thomas understood that things weren't going all that well.

"How have you been holding up?" I asked him.

I saw a flash of sadness in his eyes before he joked, "Better than the average bear!"

I validated his vibrant attitude and waited for him to share what was underneath his "everything is peachy" facade. After a few minutes his face softened, he looked at Jeremy and he audibly sighed. He shared that he hated losing his old life and his old self. He told me that he hated the fatigue most of all because he couldn't go for long walks with Jeremy like they had done every weekend for years.

"And Jeremy is your….?" It seemed clear to me that Jeremy held a special place in Thomas's life, and identifying sources of support and potential surrogate decision makers was a part of my job as a palliative care doctor.

"My roommate," Thomas said firmly.

We had a lovely chat about Thomas's work as an architect, magical trips that he and Jeremy had taken over the years, and which nurses understood his sense of humor. All my attempts to move the conversation into deeper, darker territory were met with a firm and smiling redirection.

"Is there anything that's worrying you?" I asked.

"Not really. Have you been to Greece? We loved Greece, didn't we Jeremy?" he replied.

I asked if he had an advance directive or had chosen anyone to make medical decisions for him if he ever couldn't make them for himself.

"Oh, I know I should do that. I need to make a will, too. And clean out the attic and organize my pictures. I'll get to it doc. I promise," he said.

I gave him a blank advance directive and encouraged him to fill it out before he left the hospital.

He didn't.

I saw Thomas a few months later, when his treatment had caused a problem that landed him back in the hospital. His shine was tarnished. His big personality was muted, but it wasn't gone.

"Hey, doc," he said. "Great to see you again!" he said sarcastically with a dramatic eye roll.

"It's great to see you, too," I said. "What's new?"

"I guess Jeremy's getting tired of me, so he sent me back to the hospital," Thomas said with a half-smile, glancing at Jeremy who was sitting in a chair by the window, not saying a word.

Jeremy looked tired.

I could see that Thomas was declining, and I was concerned that he still hadn't identified a medical power of attorney. Thomas wasn't married and didn't have children, so if he lost the ability to make decisions for himself it would, legally, be his two siblings who would decide what happened to him.

I tried to make my questioning sound conversational, but I had an agenda.

"What's up with your family?" I asked. "Do you see them much?"

"My brother is an a**hole and my sister keeps trying to get me to accept Jesus, so no . . . I don't see them at all," he told me.

Uh-oh.

Thomas was a strong and independent man who liked things the way he liked them. He wasn't seeing that if he didn't complete a living will and assign a medical power of attorney, the very end of his life would be utterly out of his control. And the controllers, his a**hole brother and proselytizing sister, might not choose for him what he would choose for himself.

I gave the little speech that I'd given hundreds of times.

"Advance directives are extremely important, and everyone should have one. I have one, my husband has one, and even both of my young adult daughters have one. An advance directive has two parts—a living will and a medical power of attorney. The living will part says what you would want in the future if you were near to death or weren't expected to ever wake up again. The medical power of attorney states who you would want to speak for you to the doctors if you couldn't speak for yourself. That person would make medical decisions for you if you ever couldn't make them on your own."

Thomas took a deep breath and looked at Jeremy. He didn't say a word.

Everyone should have an advance directive, but for Thomas it was a palliative care emergency that he didn't have one. Although Thomas had never said so, I had a feeling that Jeremy was his person. The person he had spent his life with, sharing adventures and hardships, and the person who should be speaking for him as this chapter of Thomas's life wrapped up.

Yet if Thomas didn't act, it wouldn't be Jeremy who would be deciding about breathing tubes and CPR and artificial feeding. It would be two people who shared Thomas's DNA but not his worldview.

I gave Thomas another blank advance directive and nearly begged him to fill it out before he left the hospital.

He didn't.

The next time I saw Thomas he was different. His cheeks were hollowed out and his skin was sallow. The twinkle in his eyes was a flicker now. Jeremy's body was folded and sagging, and his eyes were wide with fear. Everyone knew what was happening, but no one was talking about it.

As the palliative care physician, it was my job to 'go there.' To say the scary words and raise the scary topics and do everything in my power to make Thomas's time on Earth as free from suffering as possible.

"Thomas . . . what's your impression of what's happening for you?" I asked.

I saw Jeremy's eyes fill up with tears.

"Well . . . I guess it's not great," Thomas said.

I nodded but didn't say anything. Sometimes silence allows truth to bubble up.

After a while, Thomas looked at Jeremy and said, "Thank you for a wonderful life."

My eyes filled up, too.

I sat motionless as Thomas and Jeremy looked at each other and a lifetime of love and memories filled the room. I didn't wipe my tears as they spilled over onto my cheeks because I didn't want to break the spell.

Thomas spoke first. "So, what now, doc?"

"Let's talk about how you're feeling now and let's plan for the future, okay?" I asked.

"Sure, doc," he said. "Let's do it."

The veil was lifted and now we all "went there" together. We talked about dying and Thomas reassured Jeremy that he was sad, but he wasn't afraid. He made it clear that he wanted to die at home surrounded by the memories of his life and that he didn't ever want to go to the intensive care unit. If his fate was inevitable despite all intensive medical efforts, he wanted to transition to whatever was next from the comfort of his own bed.

This time I wasn't subtle.

"If that is what you want, you have to fill out this advance directive *right now*," I said in my doctor voice. It might have been closer to my mommy voice.

Thomas thought that it was good enough that he had shared the information with me and Jeremy, unwitnessed by anyone else. I knew otherwise. Officially, Jeremy was his "roommate," and no doctor was going to call on his roommate to make serious medical decisions in a life-threatening situation. In Maryland, where we were having this conversation, even I couldn't assure that Thomas's wishes got followed unless his statements were witnessed by another person. The idea of Jeremy watching powerlessly as Thomas's brother or sister overruled his wishes made my heart hurt.

"I know you don't want to think about this," I said to Thomas, "let alone talk about it, but I need you to tell me who you would want to make your medical decisions if you couldn't make them for yourself. Who knows you best? Who knows what you would want?"

"Jeremy knows me best," he said quietly.

"Would you want Jeremy to make your medical decisions for you?" I asked gently.

Thomas looked up at Jeremy, but the look was different this time. He seemed somehow smaller, and his eyes were pleading. "Would you do that for me?" he asked.

"I would do anything for you," Jeremy said with resolve.

The energy in the room had changed. Thomas could finally relax as Jeremy owned his power. Thomas had been trying to protect Jeremy from pain, but his jolly façade in the face of an unstoppable illness had had an unintended effect. Thomas's refusal to lean on Jeremy for support had left Jeremy feeling powerless and alone, as though he had been watching Thomas's decline through the window but couldn't get inside. Now Jeremy sat straighter, and his voice was strong.

"What do we need to do now, Dr. Chiaramonte?" Jeremy asked.

I pulled the paperwork out of my pocket and started filling it out. I made an X where Thomas's signature went and asked him to read the document while I popped out to get a nurse who could witness the signing of his advance directive.

I've never forgotten Thomas and Jeremy.

I've never forgotten them because that night Thomas's blood pressure dropped. His physicians were poised to call the intensive care unit and transfer him up there for tubes and medicines and machines. They called the decision-maker listed in his medical power of attorney document, Jeremy, for guidance.

Jeremy told them firmly, "Thomas wants to die in his own bed. I'm taking him home."

And that is what he did.

Thomas died two days later, surrounded by the people and the things that he loved.

The small act of completing a medical power of attorney form allowed Jeremy, the man who had adored Thomas for years, to bravely and lovingly fulfill his beloved's very last wish.

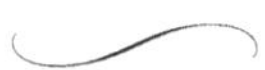

Does your loved one have a completed advance directive? Do you?

Creating an accurate and effective advance directive is a misunderstood process that is generally done poorly and without sufficient information or deep consideration. A bad advance directive may be worse than no advance directive at all.

Rose had a bad advance directive.

Rose was in her late eighties when she had a devastating stroke. She wasn't responding to her name or even to pain, and the CT scan of her head explained why. A clot had blocked off the blood flow to a huge part of Rose's brain. Her affected brain tissue was dead or dying, and although she was breathing and her heart was beating, she couldn't do much else. Her neurologist thought the chance that she would ever wake up again was less than 10 percent. The chance that Rose would ever be Rose again was closer to zero percent.

We invited her frightened son to a family meeting. He was her only relative, so it was his job to speak on his mom's behalf.

"She wouldn't want this," he told us in a sad and quiet voice.

He became animated as he told us more about his mom.

"She was a force!" he said. "She took care of everyone. She sang and danced around the house, and she was the most independent woman you'll ever meet! She would never want to live like this. Never. That woman in that bed is not my mom."

He confirmed that his mom had cared for an aging relative and, after seeing the man wither away slowly, she had made her son promise that when it was her time to go, he wouldn't try to prolong her life with a bunch of machines and tubes.

We, the medical team, confirmed that Rose's son was her healthcare surrogate and had the right to make decisions for his mom. He decided that we would not pursue CPR if her heart stopped or put a tube in her throat and hook her up to a breathing machine if she became unable to breathe on her own. He was certain that she would not want her life artificially prolonged with a feeding tube if the doctors didn't think she'd ever regain consciousness. He was clearly a loving son who had his mom's best interests at heart. We were happy that he was making tough decisions that seemed to be consistent with her wishes.

Then he found her advance directive.

Usually, it's a good thing when a family member shows up with a patient's signed advance directive, but in this case it was tragic. When a living will is done properly, it accurately reflects what a patient wants and helps the medical system to preserve people's dignity as their health declines. When it is done poorly, without guidance, it becomes a tyrant that forces everyone to do what no one wants.

Rose had filled out her advance directive at her attorney's office. Many people, unfortunately, fill out this crucial medical document with the guidance of a lawyer rather than a physician. Rose's story is a cautionary tale.

When I saw Rose's living will my heart sank. While she had chosen her son as her medical power of attorney, she had made two other crucial decisions that were about to change her life, and not in a good way.

There is an option in many advance directives to decide if your medical power of attorney has any flexibility to implement your wishes. This option exists because no one has a crystal ball. I might say that if I'm near death I don't want to be kept alive by a breathing machine, but if I'm suddenly struck by lightning and the doctors think they can get me all the way back to my normal self, please sign me up for a breathing tube. A good advance directive gives guidance but also chooses a medical power of attorney who knows you deeply enough to make the same decision that you would make if you woke up suddenly and could direct the doctors yourself. And, importantly, it gives that person some flexibility to assess the situation and tell the doctors what you would want them to do.

No one told Rose about that.

Rose's advance directive stated that she didn't want CPR or a breathing tube if she were near to death, but she *did* want a feeding tube. And she did not give her son any flexibility to modify that direction.

Here's what that meant for Rose.

Against the wishes of her son, and seemingly inconsistent with her stated wish to him that she wouldn't want her life prolonged with a bunch of tubes, Rose was on her way to getting a tube placed in her stomach so she could be fed from a bag for the rest of her life. She would be transferred to a nursing home where she would almost certainly remain unconscious and bedbound. She would be at high risk of aspiration pneumonia and bedsores. Eventually, likely months to years after her stroke, an infection would probably end her suffering by ending her life.

Her son was incredulous.

"How can you do this to her?!" He wasn't yelling but I could tell that he wanted to. "She wouldn't want to live this way. Stuck in a bed? Never waking up? I know that's not what she meant when she filled out that stupid paper."

I completely agreed with him. He had initially made the tough but loving choice to enroll his mom in hospice after her stroke and prepare for her to leave his life. But now we wouldn't, we couldn't, let him make that decision even though we all believed that that's exactly what she would have wanted.

I talked to the hospital's legal department to see if there was any way that we could let her son choose what he thought Rose would want. There wasn't. The hospital felt obligated, given what was in Rose's advance directive, to place a feeding tube and that was that.

Let me be clear: I want you, and everyone that you love, to have an accurate and clear advance directive. I want it to reflect your wishes, match your goals, and name a person who can speak for you almost as well as you can speak for yourself. What I don't want for you is a signed document that derails your end-of-life care and forces compassionate clinicians to do things to you that no one thinks you would want.

Creating a great advance directive is important and it isn't hard (see box below).

Creating a Great Advance Directive

- Fill out both parts of the advance directive: the medical power of attorney and the living will.
- Name a medical power of attorney who is willing and able to make decisions for you the way you'd make them for yourself. Be sure to ask the person if they are willing to serve.
- Talk to your medical power of attorney about what is most important to you in your life. For example, is living every single day on Earth the most important thing, or is it most important for you to be awake and able to interact with your family?
- Tell your medical power of attorney what you'd want if you were close to death or never expected to wake up again. Would you want to be kept alive with a breathing machine? Would you want to have your life artificially prolonged with a feeding tube if that meant living longer while remaining unconscious and bedbound?
- Assuming that you trust your medical power of attorney to follow your wishes, give them flexibility to make the best decision for you.
- If you have any significant change in your health, have a new discussion with your medical power of attorney.
- Revisit your advance directive once a year to be sure it still matches your wishes.
- Keep a copy in your home—don't have the only copy at your attorney's office where no one can access it if you suddenly get ill.
- Give a copy of the advance directive to your medical power of attorney, your physicians, the hospital system where you are likely to be admitted and tell others in your family where you keep your own copy.

Remember that if anyone needs to use your advance directive it means that something catastrophic has happened. Advance directives generally speak to three possible circumstances:

- You are in a persistent vegetative state

- You have an end stage illness

- You are near to death

My advance directive says that I do not want intubation or CPR if I have an end-stage illness, like advanced and untreatable cancer, but if I have a car crash tomorrow, when I'm reasonably healthy, I certainly want aggressive medical care. Pound on my chest and hook me up to the breathing machine if you think you can get me back to who I am today.

What an advance directive is really asking is, "if we think that we may not be able to bring you all the way back to who you are today, do you want us to use all the aggressive medical tools that we have, even if you might end up stuck in a bed, or hooked up to a breathing machine, for the rest of your life?"

There is no right answer to this question. Everyone is different. Personally, if I'm never expected to wake up again, I am ready to move on to whatever is after this life. But there are plenty of people who want to live every last possible minute, no matter what that looks like. Good for them. People come in different flavors, and that's beautiful. The goal of an advance directive is to communicate clearly which flavor you've chosen.

Do you want to hear one of my least favorite sentences? It is, "I don't know what she would have wanted, we never talked about it."

Every time I hear this it makes me sad. Being forced to make complicated medical decisions for someone that you love, when you have no idea what they would want, is a particular kind of unnecessary hell.

Newsflash: we're all going to die one day. Even you. Even your loved ones. Even me. All of us. Everyone. It's just part of the deal.

Do we really think that not talking about it means it won't happen? That somehow if we don't draw attention to ourselves, death might just pass us by forever? Good luck with that. I haven't seen it work so far.

Here's what I have seen:

- Young adult children terrified to make the wrong decision for their parent because the parent never told them what they would want near the end of life

- Seriously ill people denied the right to a peaceful death at home because their loved ones didn't know what to do, and doing more seemed easier than doing less

- Complicated grief after accepting intubation for a loved one who was clearly at the end of life, and then seeing that the process was more brutal than expected

- Families unable to grieve together because only a few visitors are allowed at a time in the ICU

- Loved ones making the painful choice to turn off a ventilator, which can be more emotionally fraught than avoiding it in the first place

Let's just talk about it, okay? Talking about end-of-life issues doesn't make the end-of-life come faster or bring a hex on your family. It's just an awkward thing that we don't want to talk about, but we should talk about it anyway. People talk about periods and wet dreams and erectile dysfunction. They talk about depression and suicidal feelings and wanting a divorce. I'm not saying it's fun, I'm saying you should do it even though you don't want to.

Talk to your loved one about their wishes. Be sure they fill out an advance directive if they are still able. And then talk to your family about your own wishes, too.

If you're feeling unsure about how to get started, here are some ideas:

- Have an advance directive party. Gather the family and have everyone fill out their advance directives together. If it fits your family vibe, you could have music and cake.

- Google 'advance directive' and your state and you will likely find a printable document. Go through it with your loved ones and use the document as a discussion guide.

- Watch a movie about someone near the end-of-life and use it as a springboard to talk about your loved one's wishes.

- Watch a TED talk on talking about end-of-life issues.

- Read this chapter to your loved one.

If you want more support and resources, visit my website at www. CopingSupport.com.

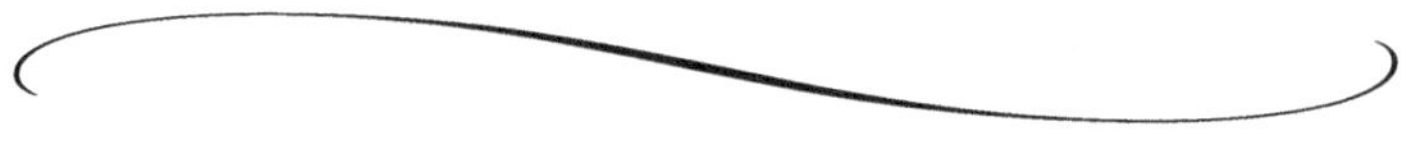

IDEA TO PONDER

How does our family handle challenging conversations?

FAMILY DISCUSSION QUESTION

What is most important to you in your life?
(Connecting with family? God? Knowledge? Nature?
Helping others? Love? Etc., etc.)

EXERCISE

Print out an advance directive for you and one for your loved one (if they are still able to complete one). Go through the document out loud and discuss each section openly. Fill out the documents and give a copy to the medical power of attorney.

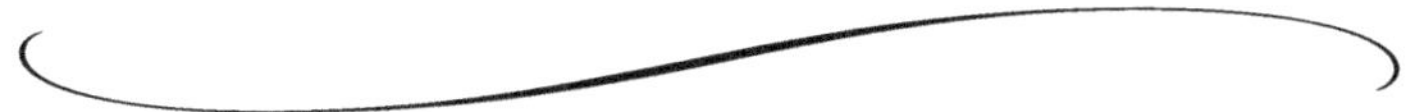

CHAPTER 5

Accept Like a Badass

I had been Nick's doctor for more than a year. He usually came to the office with his girlfriend, Nina, who kept a notebook with questions for Nick's doctors in her purse. Nina was on top of everything. She knew which chemotherapies Nick had tried and what the side effects had been. She kept track of his pain and his nausea, and she usually had a question about a potential treatment that she had researched on the internet. We used to joke that she was an honorary nurse or doctor. Nick adored her.

This day, Nick came to his appointment alone. When I saw him in the exam room, I was thrilled. Vastly different from the last time I'd seen him, this time his posture was straight, and his voice was strong. He looked robust. Nick's advanced cancer was obviously responding to his new treatment. He looked great, and he seemed to be feeling like his old self again.

"Dr. C, can I tell you a secret?" he asked me excitedly.

"Of course!" I said.

"Once I'm clear for a full year, I'm going to propose to Nina."

He looked at me expectantly. I wonder if I disappointed him, because I have no idea what came across on my face. Two powerful thoughts collided in my head all at once.

"That's wonderful!" and "Don't wait a year."

I took a moment to decide how to respond. I started with the obvious.

"I'm so happy for you. This is fantastic news. She is a wonderful woman and you're lucky to have her in your life. She's lucky too," is what I said. I wholeheartedly believed it all.

The next part was harder.

"So . . . tell me about waiting a year," I started gingerly.

He had a clear answer.

"I don't want her to marry me and then have to deal with me dying," he said.

"I get that," I said. "Will waiting a year to propose take away the risk that she'll have to deal with you dying?"

He took a deep breath. I focused on his puffed-out cheeks and the noise his breath made as it passed his pursed lips. I felt badly that I'd injected this painful reality into his good news, but I knew that it was important that we talk about his future.

"No," Nick said. "It won't. But it would make me feel better if I could just get through a whole year."

Nick had been riding a roller coaster. He'd been down then up then down then up more times than seemed fair. He had been near death and then responded to a new medication and then just as he was feeling normal again, a new pain would start or a concerning spot would show up on his imaging. His cancer had returned, not once, but over and over and over. He was sick of it.

"I totally get it, Nick," I said. "You've been through it, and you deserve some time to just be normal."

It struck me that Nick was mixing up two powerful ideas that deserved to be considered separately. Firstly, he was hoping for at least a year without a cancer recurrence. This was a reasonable hope and everyone in his life was hoping for it, too. Secondly, he had decided that he wanted to marry Nina. It was the overlap of these two goals that was causing me concern.

The chance that Nick's cancer would be permanently cured was close to zero. Barring a miracle or not-yet-invented medication, Nick's cancer would almost certainly eventually take his life. He was young. It wasn't fair.

"I don't want Nina to be a widow," Nick blurted out.

I nodded and we sat in silence for a while.

"If it comes to that . . . ," I started. "Do you think Nina would rather be a widow, losing her husband, or a woman whose boyfriend died?"

"Wow," Nick said, nodding. "I never thought about it that way. I never ever thought about it like that. I know she thinks I'm going to be cured, but . . . I think she'd rather lose her husband than her boyfriend."

"Yeah," I replied. "I think so too."

Nick and I both smiled. I felt pretty sure that he'd propose soon, and I think he started planning his proposal right there in that exam room.

I was thrilled to receive the invitation to Nick and Nina's wedding. I was proud of Nick for accepting his reality and speeding up his proposal. It would have been easier to look away, refusing to accept that a recurrence-free year was unlikely. Instead, Nick bravely accepted what he was facing and romantically asked Nina to become his wife.

Their wedding was beautiful and moving and I was honored to be invited.

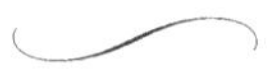

Gloria painted rocks.

She made funny rocks, rocks with colorful mandalas, and rocks with words that sparked her soul. Her rocks made her feel light, she told me, and they were a window into her spirit. They were a meditation, for her as she painted them, and for her friends and loved ones who were lucky enough to receive one. I have three of Gloria's rocks on my desk and I feel her peaceful and vibrant energy whenever I look at them.

I started my first visit with Gloria in my standard way.

"Hi. I'm Dr. Chiaramonte. Welcome to the Integrative Palliative Medicine program."

She responded with, "I want to do this right."

That wasn't typically how my patients started their visits, so I was intrigued.

I leaned in. "Tell me more about that."

"I know all about this palliative care thing," Gloria said. "I'm here because I want to do it right."

A pile of words tumbled out.

"I have ovarian cancer and I'm trying to live but I imagine it will get me eventually. I've looked it up. I know the odds. I'm going to do my best, but I don't want to be one of those people who pretends it isn't happening. I want to look it in the face and stand up tall and do what has to be done. Does this make sense? Am I crazy? I just want to do it right."

I let some silence blossom before I spoke. I wasn't sure if Gloria was expressing anxiety, perfectionism, or acceptance, and I imagined it was probably a brave and scary soup of all three. I wasn't clear on what she most needed from me, so I reflected back what I'd heard.

"So, you understand that your ovarian cancer is advanced and can't be cured. You're going to do treatment, but if there comes a time that your treatment doesn't work anymore, you're ready to accept that and face it head on. Did I get that right?"

Something shifted in the room. Gloria's forehead softened. Her lips parted and her jaw unclenched. Her shoulders drooped, but not in sad or giving up way. It was more like a weight that she had been tensing to support got lifted up and away.

"Yes" she said. "Yes."

I was inspired by Gloria's eyes wide open approach.

She stood bravely in the complexity of it all. She held herself with a strong back and an open heart. She adored her husband, her kids, her graceful dogs, and the beautiful view from her porch; she desperately wanted to live. Yet, she took nothing for granted. She practiced gratitude daily and she appreciated each moment, even the sad ones. She was able to fully embody the joy of her life and still let in the reality of her disease. She managed to stand with one foot in each world. Gloria was gloriously alive and also courageously facing the reality of her death. I was struck by her clear-eyed acceptance of what was coming alongside her fierce engagement in this beautiful world.

Acceptance gets a bad rap. In the serious illness world, it gets mixed up with giving up or not fighting or being depressed or not caring. Acceptance is painfully misunderstood. It isn't weak and it doesn't make you a quitter; it is brave and tough and fierce. Acceptance looks the monster in the eye, puffs out its chest, and says, "Yeah, I see you."

Acceptance is badass.

When people can't breathe on their own, they may be intubated. This means that a tube is placed into their airway, and it's connected to a machine that does the breathing for them. Sometimes they get better, regaining the ability to breathe on their own, and the breathing tube may be removed. This is called extubation. These people are the lucky ones.

Some people who are intubated are never able to breathe on their own again. If this is due to a traumatic injury or progressive neurologic illness, such as amyotrophic lateral sclerosis (ALS), some people choose to live their lives permanently connected to a breathing machine.

Usually, a tracheostomy tube is inserted into the trachea through an opening in the neck, and the person breathes through this tube instead of through their nose and mouth. This tube can be connected to a breathing machine, including the portable kind that can be hooked onto a wheelchair.

There is a third group of people.

These people are so ill that they cannot be weaned off a breathing machine, and they either do not want to live their life unable to breathe on their own or they are so sick that they are unlikely to live much longer with or without assisted breathing. Some patients, or families, in this circumstance choose to turn off the breathing machine and remove the breathing tube. This is called compassionate extubation, or sometimes terminal extubation. The assumption in compassionate extubation is that once the breathing tube is removed, the person's life will most likely soon be over.

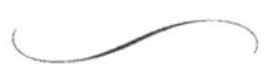

I once got called to the intensive care unit for a planned compassionate extubation.

Often there are tearful family members at the bedside. Sometimes they look lost and numb. Usually, the patient is sedated or unconscious. Not this time.

When I slid the glass intensive care unit door open, I was surprised to see Mr. M fully awake, with bright, piercing eyes. He caught my gaze and neither of us looked away. Mr. M was clearly aware of what was happening to him.

There was a tube protruding from his mouth, connected to a humming machine that was breathing for him because he could not manage this life-sustaining act on his own. He was unable to speak because of the tube in his airway, but he communicated, nonetheless. Mr. M's wife was rubbing his hand methodically. She looked terrified.

"I'm Dr. Chiaramonte from palliative care," I said as I took his other hand.

I was used to talking to families in this situation but having the patient wide awake was a new experience for me. I found it unsettling. It was hard to know what to say.

"Your doctors asked me to come see you because your condition is very serious," I started.

His eyes never unlocked from mine, and he nodded in understanding.

"They don't think you will ever be able to breathe on your own without this machine. Do you understand what I'm saying?" I asked him.

He nodded and tears spilled from the corner of his eyes. I wiped my own eyes and took a deep breath.

"Do you want us to keep this tube in your throat?" I asked him.

He very clearly shook his head, "no."

I tried a different way to be sure he understood. "Do you want us to take out the breathing tube?"

He nodded, "yes."

His wife spoke in a clear, resolved voice. "He always made me promise that I wouldn't keep him on a machine. We talked about it. I know what he wants."

I asked again, "If we take out this tube your doctors think that you will probably die. Do you understand what I'm saying?"

He didn't look away or flinch. He was steely-eyed. He looked determined and certain as he slowly nodded his head, "yes."

"Do you want us to remove this breathing tube?"

He nodded, "yes."

"Do you want us to do it today?"

He nodded, "yes."

And so, we did.

Mr. M's body was coming to an end, but his spirit was fierce. I was struck by his wholehearted and brave acceptance of what was in front of him. In no way did he give up. He faced his opponent with power and courage, right up until the end. He left this planet on his own terms.

Mr. M was tough.

He was fierce.

He was a badass.

Acceptance of death is one kind of acceptance, but there are endless other hurdles, detours, and shoe pebbles that we will all confront in our time on Earth. Developing a healthy relationship with acceptance is a skill that we all need, yet few of us have.

Let's break it down.

There is a massive misunderstanding about what acceptance is, at its core. Acceptance is not the opposite of fighting. Acceptance is the opposite of pretending.

If Gloria had rejected the reality that her cancer was progressing, she might have lost the opportunity to take a special trip, share her feelings with her loved ones, have meaningful conversations with her children, and fully review her beautiful life.

One fabulous patient of mine, a kindly woman in her sixties, bought a brand new shiny red car as her disease progressed. It was a sports car. She showed me a picture of it, and we laughed and laughed.

"Can you believe it?" she asked me. "Me, driving a sports car?" She giggled. "But really, if not now, when?"

I completely saw her point and I love that she bought that car.

Accepting what is in front of you gives you the power to choose how you want to show up for this part of life. It does not mean giving up. That's worth saying one more time. Acceptance is absolutely, one thousand percent, not giving up. It is the opposite, really.

Acceptance is looking the beast right in the eye and saying loudly and clearly, "I see you!"

Life will give you many opportunities to practice acceptance. Babies leave us for kindergarten and then college and then they get their own apartment. Beloved pets die and we lose jobs, spouses, friends, or the dream of having a biological child. Sometimes people lose a breast or a leg or a uterus or a dream.

Acceptance is a kind of spiritual practice. Clear-eyed vision is a more powerful position from which to face life's struggles than pulling the covers over your head and mumbling "lalalalalalala."

Don't shy away from acceptance because you are confusing it with giving up. Also, practicing acceptance of a difficult situation does not mean that the Universe will heap more of it upon you and break your back with the weight of it all. I believe that the reverse is true. It takes a supreme amount of energy to keep the covers over your face or bury your head ostrich-style. Also, it doesn't work. The thrumming of your fear will continue to get louder and louder.

Facing that fear or unpleasantness head-on can be a huge relief. Acceptance usually begets lightness. Once you are looking your reality clearly in the face, you can loosen your tension just a little, because it is often a bit less overwhelming than you imagined. It takes much more from you to keep it locked in the basement than it does to bring it into the light.

There is a subtlety here that is important. The goal is to accept the reality that is in front of you; the straight up, ugly, warts and all reality. My daughter could die in a car accident. Your mom might die of cancer. But we aren't mind-readers, and we can't see the future, so we don't know what *will* happen. Acceptance does not mean fortune telling. It is the acceptance of what is true, but there is always room for the Universe or God or chance, depending on your belief system, to take the story in a different direction. We are not predetermining the outcome by practicing acceptance. Instead, we are standing tall and gazing at our challenge with clear eyes and a brave heart.

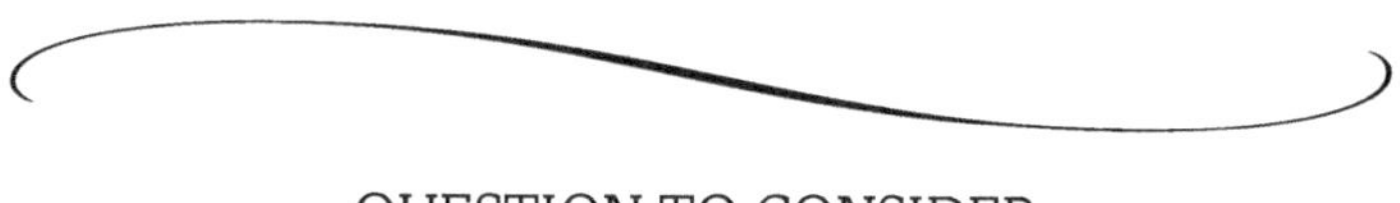

QUESTION TO CONSIDER

What does the phrase "Acceptance is not the opposite of fighting. Acceptance is the opposite of pretending" mean to you?

FAMILY DISCUSSION QUESTION

Is there anything that we should work on accepting?

EXERCISE

Make a list of at least twenty things that you could practice accepting. They can be big (a tough diagnosis) and small (graying hair or emerging wrinkles).

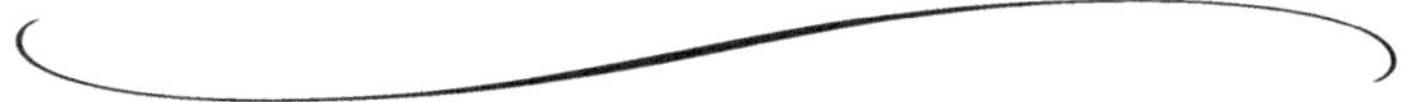

CHAPTER 6

Create an Imperfect Plan

Nancy had been a powerhouse when she was younger. She'd been a dancer, had socialized in exclusive circles, and had traveled the world with her husband. Her children wouldn't have described her as the perfect mother, but they had never gone hungry, and the family was still reasonably close. Since her husband had died several years before, Nancy, at eighty-one, had lived alone. She read voraciously and enjoyed tending her garden and watching the cardinals and finches that frequented her bird feeder. She talked to each of her three daughters once a week, chatting about the news, books she'd read, or small family dramas. She rarely complained, and her daughters assumed that everything was fine.

Her daughters didn't know that Nancy sometimes put the wrong pills into the slots of her pillbox or took too many of one medication and too few of another. Nancy never mentioned that she'd once accidentally left the stove on all day. Her daughters didn't know that sometimes Nancy woke up and couldn't figure out where she was.

One morning, Nancy's daughter, Mary, called to check in. Something didn't seem right.

"Are you okay, mom?" Mary asked.

"I'm okay. It's okay. You're okay," Nancy said.

"Mommy, is something wrong?" Mary asked again, feeling a tightness in her throat.

She started looking for her keys.

Mary drove the hour to her mother's house with stinging eyes and tightness in her chest. When she got there, she found Nancy wandering around the apartment, clearly disoriented. She took her immediately to the emergency department.

When the doctors asked her to tell them the date and where she was, Nancy had been baffled. She could only tell them her name.

Mary was shaken. She'd never seen her mother like this.

"What is happening to her?" Mary asked the doctor. She didn't wait for him to answer. "You can fix this, right?" she asked with wide eyes and a constricted voice. "You have to fix this."

"I'll do my best," the doctor said.

Mary was not reassured.

"What if mom can't come home?" she wondered with rising panic. "I can't take her home with me," Mary thought. "I just can't do it."

Just thinking about this made Mary feel sick. She loved her mom and felt terrible about not wanting to move her in. But Mary's life was overfull already and she couldn't imagine how it would work.

She and her sisters had never discussed what they would do if Nancy couldn't live alone anymore. Occasionally, one of them had mentioned that they should talk to her about it, but time passed, and it felt awkward, so they had never gotten around to it.

Mary had had her children late and she still had a few kids at home. One of her sisters worked all the time and the other one lived in a tiny apartment and was struggling just to take care of herself. But Nancy had made them promise that they'd never make her go to "the home."

Mary felt panicked.

Nancy's doctors surmised that she had taken too many of several of her medications, which had worsened her confusion. To be safe, they had also checked her for a urinary tract infection and pneumonia, but she didn't have either. The doctors presented this like it was good news, but Mary wasn't so sure. An infection could be cured. If Nancy was confusing her medications for no particular reason, this seemed like bad news to Mary.

Now, with doctors in charge of her medications, Nancy's extreme confusion cleared up. She could accurately state the date, explain where she was, and even joke around with the nurses. Still, Mary noticed that she repeated stories and didn't seem quite as sharp as she used to be.

When the doctors were ready to send Nancy home, no one mentioned any specific instructions to Mary, so she picked her mom up, took her out to lunch, and dropped her off at her apartment.

Mary felt uneasy. She didn't have words to describe the feeling, but she noticed a heaviness in her gut and a prickly sensation at the back of her neck. She promised herself that she would call her mom every day to check on her. She didn't mention any of this to her sisters because she didn't want to worry them.

For a while everything seemed okay.

Mary's new routine was to call her mom daily and visit once a week. She filled Nancy's pillbox every Sunday, made sure her fridge was stocked, and did a load of laundry. After a few months of this, Mary was exhausted.

She dropped hints to her sisters about how hard it was to balance caring for Nancy and being there for her husband and her kids. Her head was spinning as she tried to balance sports games, homework help, volunteering at school, and teenage emotions, along with caring for her mom. Forget date night or keeping the house neat and doing anything for her own well-being; those weren't even on the table anymore. She felt like she was balancing twenty spinning ceramic plates and they were all about to crash to the ground and shatter.

"You know, it would be great if you could visit mom some weekend to give me a break," she told her sister Lena. She tried not to sound annoyed.

"Okay, okay. I'll try. You know how busy I am at work, though," Lena said. "I can't just drop everything and drive two hours to make mom a sandwich."

Mary's cheeks flushed and her jaw clenched.

"Never mind. Just forget it," she told Lena.

Mary didn't even bother asking her other sister, Jenna, for help.

If you have siblings and your loved one has a serious illness, you might identify, at least a little bit, with Mary or one of her sisters.

Maybe you feel like you carry 97 percent of the burden, and your siblings don't help enough, or even at all. Or maybe you feel like your sibling acts like a martyr and always tries to make you feel guilty that you aren't doing enough. Or maybe your siblings leave you out and assume that you can't be helpful just because you are somehow outside of the family mold or live across the country.

Caring for a loved one with a serious illness can bring out the teenager in all of us. You know, the part that feels put upon, wronged, misunderstood, dismissed, or overburdened. Family illness can strain even the closest relationships.

When a parent gets ill, childhood wounds can resurface, and powerful feelings like shame, anger, and guilt can seep into family communication like a smelly, toxic gas leak. Even a tiny spark can make the whole thing blow up.

"Yes, but you don't know my brother, or sister," you might be thinking. "He's so difficult, there's no talking any sense into him."

Or "She's so selfish, she'll never help out."

Or "He's so bossy that he'll try to take over everything, even though he hasn't seen dad in two years!"

Most families have at least one challenging member. They may cause drama, be rampant complainers, or doggedly focus on the negative aspects of the situation. Perhaps they are bossy or maybe they're disengaged. The solution is not to simply be more understanding. The solution is to take a realistic assessment of everyone's needs, struggles, and abilities and consciously create an imperfect plan.

Creating An *Imperfect Plan* with Your Family

If you're thinking that you want a perfect plan, not an imperfect one, I have bad news for you. You can't have that. You can't have a perfect plan because you aren't a perfect person, and neither is anyone in your family. Everyone has wounds and idiosyncrasies and burdens and quirks and, to one degree or another, they will always have them. When life is hard or stressful or scary our quirks get quirkier, and our wounds get deeper.

Navigating a tough situation with your family members is rarely easy. Almost every family has childhood grievances that resurface, sticky personalities that get stickier under pressure, or far-away siblings who suddenly show up with strong opinions. You may be certain that you are the reasonable one and the others are the problem. You could be right. But I gently suggest that you consider the possibility that you are only partially right. Your negative emotions, fears, or prickly personality traits may bring out the worst in your people. And theirs may bring out the worst in you. This doesn't always happen, of course. Some families buoy each other when times are tough, but even in the closest of families tension can seep in.

When dealing with a loved one's illness, each person in the family, including you, may step into a persona and find it challenging to break free. One person may take on the job of martyr while others may adopt qualities such as avoider, controller, or victim. Sometimes you may all cycle through different personas at different times.

My loving advice to you is to be gentle with each other. It is likely that everyone in the family is suffering, and they are doing the best that they can at an emotionally charged and painful time.

When you encounter your sibling or parent or cousin or aunt or uncle or grandparent bringing their difficult self to the table, try to silently block their words before they reach your ears. They are allowed to be difficult, but you don't need to receive their messy or unhelpful thoughts or emotions. Try to imagine that they are speaking Swahili (that is, unless you speak Swahili, in which case you could imagine them speaking Albanian). The idea is to imagine that you can see their mouth moving but you have no idea what they are saying. Your goal is to allow them to process their negative emotions without igniting yours.

Creating your imperfect plan has three steps.

First, you will prepare yourself so that you don't inadvertently sabotage the plan with unrealistic expectations, old wounds, or unhelpful criticism. Second, you will actively use curiosity instead of expectation to brainstorm solutions. Third, you will match the helpers to the tasks that they agree to take on and unemotionally assess the gaps. I suggest that you write down your imperfect plan, give everyone involved a copy, and revisit the plan at least every few months. If your loved one has a change in their health, that is the perfect time to revisit the imperfect plan. If you'd like a template to create your imperfect plan, one is available at www.CopingSupport.com.

Let's use Mary and her family as an example.

1. Prepare Yourself

Mary is annoyed at her sisters. She feels that she has been doing all the work caring for her mom, and her sisters won't help. She assumes that they must know how overwhelmed she feels, and they obviously don't care. She thinks that they are being selfish and unsupportive and, when she isn't feeling furious at them, she has to admit that she is hurt. If they cared about her, they would help more.

Before Mary calls her family together to create an imperfect plan, it would be helpful to work on her own feelings first. People sense each other's energy, and if Mary brings that hurt and angry energy to a conversation with her sisters, they are likely to get defensive. The conversation is unlikely to be as productive as it could be. In fact, the meeting might descend into a battle of 'who is more wounded,' and their relationship could end up even more challenged than it is right now.

This does not mean that Mary must squash her own feelings or prioritize her siblings' feelings over her own. Not at all. This is simply an intentional approach to managing everyone's strong emotions in order to get your family's imperfect plan completed despite an imperfect situation.

Mary's first step in preparing herself is to acknowledge the uncomfortable feelings that are weighing her down or riling her up. She can speak them out loud to herself, tell another person, or write them in a journal. Simply thinking about them is generally not sufficient.

"I am feeling angry, hurt, scared, sad, and lonely," Mary might say to herself in the mirror.

Once you say your feelings out loud, go one level deeper. Why are you feeling that way? When have you felt that way before?

Here's what Mary might say, or write, next. "I'm feeling angry because my sisters leave the hardest things for me to deal with. I'm hurt because I feel like they don't really care about me. They've been leaving me out since we were kids. I'm scared because I have no idea what is going to happen. I'm sad because I don't want to lose my mom, and I'm lonely because it feels like I'm on a sinking ship all by myself."

Speaking her feelings out loud, or writing them in a journal, won't make them magically go away. I wish it worked that way, but removing the feelings is not actually the point of saying them out loud. Speaking your feelings out loud takes them out of the shadows and allows you to assess them with clear eyes. You can then make a plan, both short term and long term, to address them. Actively managing your strong feelings makes them much less likely to hijack your family conversations.

In the long-term, Mary might choose to see a grief counselor, psychotherapist, art therapist, or religious leader to get support in dealing with her strong feelings. But what can Mary do to manage her strong emotions in the short term? How can she use her new awareness to prepare for a conversation with her siblings as they create an imperfect plan to care for their mom?

There are many possible approaches, but the underlying idea is to acknowledge and process the feelings so they lose some of their power, and then actively reduce the physiological stress response that these feelings have revved up. I suggest that you make a plan with at least three components. Try to choose an approach that allows you to both share your feelings and also reduce your stress. Here are a few ideas, but there are an unlimited number of equally valid ones that you might come up with for yourself.

Idea Number One

- Have a marathon phone call with your closest friend and talk it all out

- Take a long shower and sob until there are no more tears

- Take the dog for a walk in the woods and focus on the sights and smells of the forest

Idea Number Two

- Buy a new journal and write all about what is happening

- Arrange for weekly massages

- Spend time coloring in a grown-up coloring book every evening after dinner

Idea Number Three

- Join a support group for families with a seriously ill loved one

- Schedule a weekly acupuncture session

- Download a relaxation app and listen to a guided meditation every morning

If Mary approaches her imperfectly imperfect planning session with her siblings from a calmer and more balanced state of mind, the chance of working together successfully will markedly increase.

While Mary's newfound balance may increase the chance that her siblings will stay calm, it certainly doesn't guarantee it. It can be helpful to prepare what she will do if one of her siblings gets agitated, frustrated, or mean. The simplest approach is to imagine that the agitated person is a two-year-old who is throwing a tantrum.

When toddlers have tantrums, their words are irrelevant. All their words essentially mean the same thing: "I am in distress, and I can't handle my strong feelings." If a toddler says, "I hate you," they don't really hate you, or at least they won't hate you after a nap. If they say, "you aren't my mommy," it doesn't mean you aren't their mommy. And you will gain no benefit by trying to prove to the overwhelmed child that you are, in fact, their mommy. All the words mean the same thing: "I am in distress, and I can't handle my strong feelings."

So, if your siblings act out during a conversation about your sick loved one, they are generally communicating "I am in distress, and I can't handle my strong feelings." Try not to get sucked in by the words. "You just think you're better than the rest of us" means "I am in distress, and I can't handle my strong feelings."

"Mom always spoiled you so you've never carried your weight in the family" means "I am in distress, and I can't handle my strong feelings."

"You are so selfish" means "I am in distress, and I can't handle my strong feelings."

"You are doing this all wrong" means "I am in distress, and I can't handle my strong feelings."

The best way to handle a toddler tantrum is to ignore it. They can fuss all they want, while you sip a latte and savor a croissant. Occasionally a boundary will be needed (if they start breaking plates, for example), but other than that, the most important task is to keep yourself calm. Try to use this same approach with challenging family members. Set a boundary if things get too ugly, but otherwise ignore, ignore, ignore. Their mouth is moving but you can't understand the words.

How to keep calm in a stressful situation

- Rub your thumb and index finger together and focus on trying to feel the ridges of your fingers.
- Take three deep breaths, making the exhale longer than the inhale. Repeat as often as you need to.
- Count your breaths, saying "one" to yourself as you breathe in and "breathe" to yourself as you breathe out. Do this until you count to ten.
- Splash cold water on your face.
- Walk up and down the stairs a few times or do ten jumping jacks.
- Rub your palms together until they get warm. Focus on the sound and the feeling of warmth.
- Imagine each part of your body relaxing, starting with your forehead and progressing to your feet. As you imagine each part, focus on relaxing and softening it.

Once you have practiced acknowledging your emotions and calming your stress response, see if you can access a feeling of empathy, at least for yourself. This is a really tough situation, and you are doing your best to manage it. You aren't perfect and that's okay. If you can drum up a feeling of empathy for your family, you deserve a hundred extra points or an extra scoop of ice cream.

The last part of preparation for creating your imperfect plan is acceptance. This doesn't mean you have to accept that your loved one won't get better. Rather, you are accepting that the process of managing it all will be imperfect. You will lose your cool, your family members will be annoying, the doctors might be frustrating, and your loved one may or may not improve. Expecting perfection in such a fraught situation is a set up for increasing your distress. A little bit of "it is what it is" energy can make your journey through this imperfect process a little smoother.

Be Curious

Expectation is heavy and sets you up for disappointment, while curiosity has a lightness to it that allows new ideas to reveal themselves.

Mary currently has expectations about her sisters.

"Lena will say she's too busy and Jenna will start crying and say she can't handle it. I'll be left doing it all just like I always am," Mary might say to herself.

Mary probably has good reasons for these expectations but bringing this energy to the conversation reduces the chance of success, so it is to her benefit to approach the meeting in a new way. Mary might ask herself, "Would I rather be right, or would I rather have a productive meeting?"

If Mary were to bring a spirit of curiosity to the meeting, she might ask herself some of the following questions.

- I wonder what will help Lena and Jenna be open and calm during our meeting?

- I wonder what Lena and Jenna are feeling right now?

- I wonder what Lena will be able to contribute since she is very busy at work?

- I wonder what Jenna will want to contribute?

- I wonder if Jenna is stronger than we give her credit for?

- I wonder what I will need during this conversation to stay calm?

- I wonder what will help me ask for help and get my needs met?

- I wonder what it would take for the three of us to feel like we're on the same team?

- I wonder what would work best for Mom?

- I wonder if there is anyone else in the family who can help pay for hired care?

- I wonder if anyone at Mom's religious institution would be able to help?

- I wonder what I could get help with at home to give me more energy to deal with this situation?

- I wonder if I could let go of any of my responsibilities so I don't get so worn out and depleted?

- I wonder if my spouse could help out more?

- I wonder if I could take some time off work?

- I wonder if there is anyone else that I know who could offer some support?

- I wonder if I can model this curiosity approach for Lena and Jenna?

When we get stuck in the 'what should I do?' part of our brain, we have easy access to approaches that have worked before. But when dealing with a new and challenging situation, it can be helpful to tap into the more creative, outside-the-box part of our brain to explore new and innovative solutions.

Match Helpers to Tasks

Once you've prepared yourself for the conversation, and practiced adopting a creative spirit, you are ready to schedule your family meeting and create your imperfect plan (see box on p. 96).

During your meeting you can brainstorm all the tasks that need to be covered. For example:

- Take Dad to appointments
- Fill Mom's weekly pillbox
- Check on Dad daily
- Get groceries weekly
- Cook and freeze meals
- Schedule doctors' appointments
- Clean house and do laundry
- Pay Mom's bills
- Arrange for a neuropsychology assessment
- Have Mom fill out an advance directive
- Have Mom designate one of us as a social security payee
- Have Mom fill out a financial power of attorney form
- Etc., etc.

I suggest that you create a grid with the following labels at the top:

- Task
- Who can help
- How often
- Notes

Here's a sample helper grid:

Task	Helper	Schedule	Notes
Food shopping	Rachel	Every Saturday	No dairy
Pay Dad's bills	John	First Sunday of Month	Dad wants to help
Call to check on Dad	Anna, Rachel, John	Anna: Mon, Wed Rachel: Tues, Thurs John: Fri, Sat, Sun	If can't reach Dad after three tries, call neighbor to check on him in person

A downloadable grid is available at www.CopingSupport.com.

After you brainstorm all the things that need to be done, you're ready to have an open, honest, nonjudgmental conversation with your people. You are simply trying to identify what needs to be done and what everyone is willing and able to do. There will be gaps. Expect them. Importantly, do your absolute best not to judge who is helping more and who is helping less. At this stage, you are just trying to figure out what everyone thinks they can contribute. Some of you might be willing to visit frequently. Others might be willing to pay for hired help. Some will be willing to clean the house, while others will make all the appointments and talk to the doctors.

Don't judge.

Your brother isn't willing to visit, but he is willing to pay for food delivery. Don't judge.

Your sister will only visit once a month, but when she's there she'll clean, do laundry, and change the sheets. Don't judge.

Your aunt is only willing to stop by now and then to play cards. Don't judge.

People will do what they feel able to do. You may not agree with their choices, but you cannot change them. Some people might do nothing at all to help right now, and there's nothing you can do about that either. If this is your situation, you are likely hovering somewhere between frustrated and furious. If someone in the family doesn't help in the way that you think they should, particularly if you feel like the extra burden is falling on you, it can be maddening. You may want to shake them by the shoulders until they understand how desperately you need them to help. If that worked, I'd be all for it. The problem is, sometimes the more you try to push someone into helping more, the more firmly they dig in to helping less. The backwards reality is, often you will get the best out of potential helpers by respecting their limits and calmly collaborating on a plan. If their limits are respected now, they may decide to help more in the future. And, of course, you get to set your limits, too. What can you realistically do to help? Fill in the grid with all the tasks that need to be done and who can take on which task.

This is the first pass.

You will almost certainly have gaps.

The first question to ask the group is, "Can we pay someone to fill in these gaps?"

Perhaps someone in the family is willing to foot the bill. Maybe someone on the list will organize a fundraiser. Perhaps your loved one has the funds to cover this help. Maybe a friend, extended family member, or religious organization can provide financial assistance. Be creative. Ask, "I wonder who could help us afford to pay for this?"

If you are still left with gaps, ask "I wonder how we could fill in these gaps?"

Perhaps one of your family members will volunteer to take on a little more. Maybe you will decide to put a call out to other family members or friends to see what they can contribute. Maybe you'll investigate adult daycare programs or assisted living facilities. Maybe you'll contact a social worker or caregiving expert for advice. Every situation is different, but the spirit of curiosity and non-judgmental problem-solving works for most of them.

Anatomy of a family meeting

Before the Meeting
- Arrange a mutually agreeable time, in person or online.
- Decide who will "host" the meeting.
- Decide who will take notes and distribute them after the meeting.
- Agree on ground rules. These might include: no yelling, no name-calling, no bringing up issues from the past, no using the phrases "you always . . . " or "you never . . . ," no dominating the conversation, no interrupting, no judging, etc. Try to commit to treating each other respectfully.
- State a goal for the meeting. For example, "We are going to make a plan for keeping Mom as safe as possible at home," or "We're going to discuss the option of surgery and see if we can come to a decision about whether or not to authorize it."

During the Meeting
- Ask everyone for a thirty- to sixty-second check-in (no more). They might say, "I'm feeling a little agitated today," or "I didn't sleep well last night," or "I went for a walk this morning, so I feel pretty good," or "I'm nervous about this meeting."
- Review the ground rules.
- Restate the goals of the meeting.
- State a plan for the meeting but allow flexibility. For example, "Let's review what the doctor said and decide on what needs to be done, then everyone will have a chance to share their perspective, and then we can discuss a plan." Or "Let's write down all of the things that need to be done for Mom and figure out how each of us can help out."
- Suggest a spirit of curiosity and encourage the use of the phrase "I wonder."
- Put a sticky note or phone reminder in your line of sight that says, "don't judge."

- Discuss the meat of your meeting. Be sure everyone gets to speak. If someone hasn't spoken up, ask them to share their opinion.
- Towards the end of the allotted time, discuss whether you'll be finishing your imperfect plan during this meeting or if another meeting will be required.
- Decide how often you will review your imperfect plan.
- Schedule your next meeting.

After the Meeting:

- Send notes of the meeting to the group.
- Review your imperfect plan as scheduled and assess how it is working for your loved one and the helpers.

Newsflash! Your imperfect plan will be imperfect. This means that some of the helpers will help in a way that is not up to your standards, some will do an objectively lousy job, and others simply won't do what they promised at all. This is reality, so you might as well prepare yourself.

There are two questions to ask in this situation. One question is for you and the other is for the slacking helper. Here's your question:

Is this critical? If your sibling didn't show up to take your mom to a crucial doctor's appointment, that's a problem. But how about if they "cleaned" her apartment and left some dust bunnies behind? It might be annoying but it isn't a catastrophe. It is highly possible that some people on your helper list will complete a task in a way that you consider substandard. How should you handle this non-critical but substandard work?

Should you point out what they did wrong? Should you explain to them how you would have done it? Should you ask them to do it again?

Nope, nope, and nope. What should you do if someone adequately completes a task, but not to your satisfaction? You should take some deep breaths, jog in place for a few minutes, and then get the heck over it as soon as you can. If your sibling left a spill in the fridge, bought too much junk food, or took dad out in embarrassingly mismatched clothes, let it go. I know you would have done it better. Let it go anyway.

And this leads to the second question for your slacking helper. If the issue is, in fact, critical, you need a different approach. If Dad's pill box didn't get filled, Mom's bills weren't paid, or your elderly aunt now has bedsores because no one cleaned her up for days, that's a problem that needs to be addressed. In this case, the question for your helper is:

What are the barriers that are making it hard for you to complete your part of the imperfect plan?

If you are feeling generous you might add:

How can I help you overcome those barriers?

While it might be tempting to fuss at a helper who isn't being helpful, it is more effective to explore barriers and brainstorm solutions than it is to simply nag. Nagging rarely works, and it can drive a wedge between you and your people that can be hard to dislodge.

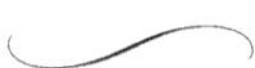

Mary and her sisters created an imperfect plan.

They determined who would visit Nancy and how often. They assigned tasks such as filling Nancy's pillbox, buying groceries, cooking food, and cleaning the house. They decided who would help Nancy fill out her medical and financial power of attorney forms and who would talk to her about her medical wishes and help her fill out her living will. They decided who would help her designate a social security payee and who would help her pay bills. They did identify some gaps, and Lena agreed to pay for hired help since she didn't feel able to visit Nancy that frequently. They divvied up daily phone calls so that Nancy would hear from one of them every day.

Creating an imperfect plan can be challenging, and the process may be bumpy. That's okay. Imperfect plans are meant to be imperfect. But if you make the effort to prepare yourself, make space for creative solutions, and nonjudgmentally match tasks with what each of you can realistically contribute, you can craft a plan that brings your family closer and keeps your loved one safer.

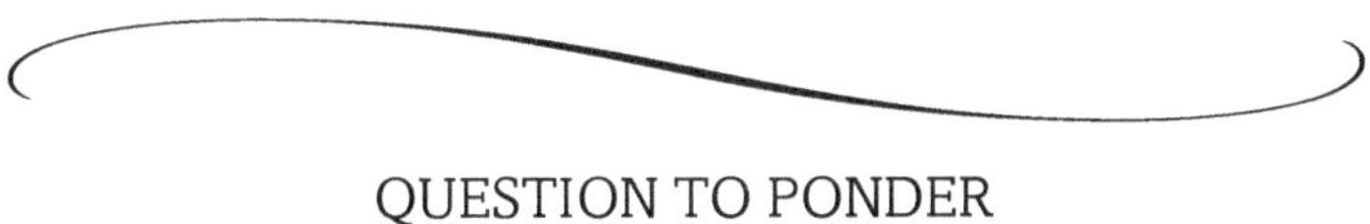

QUESTION TO PONDER

How could you prepare yourself before creating an Imperfect Plan with your family?

FAMILY DISCUSSION QUESTION

What are the strengths of everyone in the family that could be useful in an Imperfect Plan?

EXERCISE

Create an Imperfect Plan for your family.

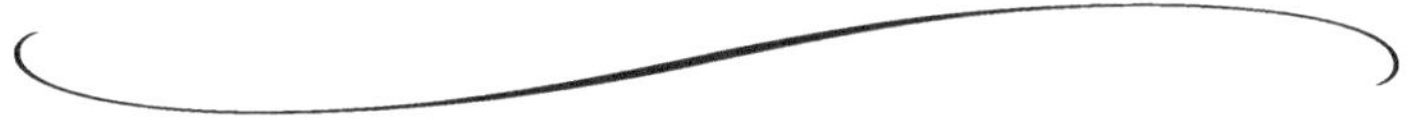

PAUSE BREAK

Place the fingers of your dominant hand on the palm of your
other hand.

Slowly and gently move your fingers over your palm.

Pay exquisite attention to the ridges and bumps on your palm.

Notice all the sensations that you feel
on your palm and on your fingers.

Switch hands.

Take one slow deep breath.

Part 2

Cultivate Growth and Build Resilience

CHAPTER 7

Control What You Can

Ellen was a sixty-one-year-old woman who was enjoying her early retirement. She had regular lunch dates with friends, played tennis every Thursday, and watched her granddaughter on Saturday mornings to give her daughter and son-in-law a break. She and her husband tried to walk two miles after dinner a few nights a week.

Life was good.

Ellen hadn't been to the gynecologist for a while, but she finally scheduled an appointment. When the day arrived, she got there early, chatted casually with the staff, changed into a flimsy paper gown, and hopped onto the exam table. She knew what was coming next and she dreaded it. She had always hated getting a Pap smear.

The doctor was friendly and funny. They laughed about how awkward pelvic exams were and they exchanged stories about their kids. Ellen tensed up when the doctor touched her, but she took some deep breaths and told herself that it would be over soon. She was relieved when the doctor finally removed the speculum. She prepared for the manual exam and reassured herself that soon she'd be dressed and heading to the coffee shop.

Then the air in the room changed.

She saw something on the doctor's face that hadn't been there before. A darkness. A focus. Ellen noticed that the doctor, with two fingers inside her vagina and a hand on her abdomen, was spending a lot of time on the right side of her pelvis.

"Is everything okay?" Ellen asked, trying to sound light and unconcerned.

"Why don't you get dressed and then we'll talk," the doctor said.

She tried to sound casual, but Ellen heard the subtext. The doctor's whole vibe had changed. Something was wrong.

Dressed and nervous, Ellen waited in the doctor's office. Her chest felt tight, and she wished her husband had come with her. Just as she was about to call him, the doctor came in. This time there was no small talk.

"One of your ovaries feels abnormal," the doctor said. "I'm concerned."

"Concerned?" Ellen repeated with her eyebrows raised and her head tilted to one side. "Concerned like 'you might need to come back for a test' or concerned like 'something bad is happening?'"

Ellen already knew the answer, deep in her gut, but she was hoping for a sliver of reassurance from the doctor. She didn't get it. The doctor was all business now. No more joking, no more family stories.

"I can't know for sure, of course, but I am concerned that you might have ovarian cancer."

Just like that, Ellen's whole world flipped upside down.

By the time she saw me, Ellen had been scanned and biopsied and the reality was clear. She had advanced, and incurable, ovarian cancer.

"How am I supposed to live my life now that I know I'm going to die?" Ellen asked.

She led with that. It was the greatest burden on her mind. She asked me again.

"Seriously, how am I supposed to go back to my life now that I know I'm going to die?"

I've been asked this question over and over. This question bubbles up in people of all ages, races, and ethnic backgrounds. It surfaces in people who are sure they know what comes after death, and in those who aren't sure there is anything at all.

"How can I live now that I know I'm going to die?"

This question is multi-layered, and it has a companion question: "How can I live now that I know my (insert beloved loved one) is going to die?"

I am of two minds when I think about this question. First, I hear anticipatory grief. The idea of losing one's space on this planet or having to say goodbye to someone that you love is brutally painful and unsettling and sad. It deserves support and counseling and prayer if that's your thing. Sometimes a good cry is in order, or journaling or snuggling with a dog on the couch. Anticipatory grief is hard. There are things that can help, and we'll talk more about that in later chapters. That said, there is another important dimension to this question. Let's look at the question one more time.

"How can I live now that I know I'm going to die?"

Do you see it?

Here is the question that I have for you: when in your life did you not know that you are going to die?

I can hear your objections already.

"No, no, no. That's not the same thing. Now I know that I'm going to die of ovarian cancer."

Do you, though? Do you know for sure what you're going to die of, even once your doctor gives you a life-limiting diagnosis? There are people with ovarian cancer who die in car accidents, people with kidney disease who die in plane crashes, and people with heart disease who fall down the stairs and don't get up again.

Let's remind ourselves of the truth: we're all going to die. You, me, and everyone that we love. The other, perhaps more unsettling, truth is that none of us have any idea when or how it will happen. Magical thinking around death is rampant. We assume that if no one has told us otherwise, we're good. We will get to stay on this floating blue ball for so long that we just won't worry about it. We think we can look around a room and pick out the guy who is going to die first. You have gray hair and walk with a cane? You're it! This gives us a comforting sense of control.

It feels so much better to believe that there is order in the world than to imagine that anything can happen at any time. Young people live and old people die, right? If I don't have cancer, I won't die but if I do have cancer I should start to worry, right? Well, . . . yes and no. Of course, having a serious illness doesn't improve your chances of not dying, but it also isn't the first time that dying has been on the table. Living indefinitely is not a prize that any of us have a prayer of winning. Dying was in your future from the moment you were conceived. And the disturbing but truly true truth is that none of us know when our number will be called. "Yes, but they're so young," or "she takes such good care of herself," or "he plays tennis twice a week," you might say with your magical thinking hat on. None of it matters. We die when our number is up, and none of us know what our number is or when it will be called.

Ironically, fully immersing yourself in the reality that life is fragile and every day is a gift that we are not promised is key to thriving when a serious illness comes into your world.

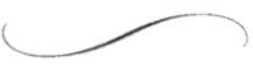

I don't want to die.

I assume that you don't want to die, either.

Yet we have all, for much of our lives, perfected the skill of both knowing that we will die one day and somehow not knowing it at the same time. We put the idea of our eventual death so far back in our metaphorical closet, behind the clothes that will never fit again and the swim fins from when we went scuba diving that one time, that it rarely enters our awareness.

So how do you live now that you know you're going to die? The same way you have for your entire life. You do what needs to be done (wear your seatbelt, look both ways when you cross the street, show up for chemo, get your colonoscopy) and then you put that thought on a shelf and go out to lunch. In other words, you know it, but you intentionally don't spend much time looking at it. Imagine if every morning before you drove to work you spent an hour looking on the internet for car accident statistics and vividly imagined yourself dying in a blazing crash. Then every night as you waited for sleep, you imagined how your family would get the news and how they would feel looking at the pictures of the wrecked car. Can you imagine? If you did that every day for even a week you would be a mess. Please do not do this. Here's what you should do instead:

Control what you can and let go of the rest.

I'm certainly not saying you should have a vodka soda before speeding to work in your car without your seatbelt on. This would not be a good plan. You should wear your seatbelt, drive the speed limit, avoid the urge to text in the car, and pay close attention to the road. This is within your control. But there is something that you shouldn't do. You should not spend the whole ride thinking about car crashes. Ruminating about dying in a car accident does not make you safer, in fact it may distract you and make you less safe, and it will markedly increase your distress. Am I saying that you will not die in a car crash if you wear your seatbelt and drive the speed limit? Nope. I wish I could promise you that. You could do all the right things and still have a lousy outcome. That's just the way the world works.

It may sound like I'm suggesting more things for you to be worried about, but I'm not. Well, I am suggesting more bad things that could happen; however, there are so many tragic things that *could* happen to us, an infinite number of unimagined things, that there is simply no value in picking a specific thing to worry about. And there simply isn't time in the day to actively worry about all the terrible things that could happen, so I propose another approach.

What if we actively avoided worrying about any of them?

I have lived this plan myself.

My first baby cried all the time. I mean *all the time*. All day, all night, and especially every time she ate. She had watery poop and was covered in a rash, but her pediatrician wasn't worried so neither was I. I wasn't concerned, but I was exhausted.

My baby would start to breastfeed but then scream and writhe and pull away and I wasn't sure what to do. The pediatrician told me not to worry, so I called a lactation consultant to help me figure out what I was doing wrong. I was a brand-new mom and I figured there were tricks to breastfeeding that I just hadn't figured out yet. It turns out that I wasn't the problem.

"Your baby has food allergies," she said definitively. "I want you to take dairy, wheat, eggs, nuts, sesame, soy, and seafood out of your diet, and then we'll see what happens."

I did as I was told. I even gave up my favorite treat, peanut butter on a sesame bagel. It was miraculous. Someone took away my screaming, rashy, liquid pooping, non-breastfeeding baby and replaced her with a clear-faced one who slept, ate, and filled her diapers with normal stuff. Just for the heck of it, I went back to my usual diet for a few days to see what would happen. You can imagine what happened. Clearly, if I wanted my daughter to feel better, I needed to stop feeding her foods that made her sick, so I stopped drinking milk, gave up eggs, and learned to eat without any of the major allergens.

Things went great for a while. She grew out of her milk allergy and passed her peanut challenge at age two. We celebrated with pizza and ice cream and put the epi pens, which we happily no longer needed, in the back of a cabinet.

We sent her to preschool at age four without worry. When the school nurse called me one day in the middle of what would normally be nap time, I assumed that my daughter had a fever or had thrown up her lunch.

"Something is happening, Delia, but we don't want you to worry," the nurse said. "Your daughter was making peanut butter bird feeders with her class and now she says her throat feels funny and she has a rash."

"Is she wheezing or coughing?" I asked with an escalating feeling of panic. I knew that about 30,000 food-allergic people end up in the emergency department with anaphylaxis every year, and a couple hundred of them die. It seemed that my daughter's nut allergy had returned, and she was having a significant allergic reaction. Coughing or wheezing would be a dangerous and scary sign.

"Yes," the nurse said matter-of-factly.

I found my calm doctor voice. "Do you have an EPIPEN® at the school?" I asked.

This injectable treatment for anaphylaxis can be lifesaving for someone having a severe allergic reaction, and my daughter needed an injection of epinephrine right away.

"No," the nurse replied without any apparent concern.

"Please call 911 immediately and I will be there as soon as I can," I said.

To my surprise, the nurse argued with me. "Is that really necessary?" she asked in a snidely rhetorical way designed to make me sound alarmist and dramatic.

"Yes. It is," I said firmly.

When I told her that I would call the paramedics myself and send them to the school if she refused to get my daughter the appropriate medical care that she needed, she finally relented.

This experience was the start of a journey that trained me to increase my focus on what I could control and let go of what I couldn't.

Food-allergic children who also have asthma are more likely to die. My daughter has asthma. In the beginning, I could not stop thinking about this. How was I supposed to send her back to school, where baked goods and candy were firmly integrated into the culture, when I couldn't be there to administer a life-saving epinephrine injection? She was too young to be trusted to stay away from unsafe but yummy goodies, and the teachers seemed to think that I was just an anxious mom. I hoped for vigilance, but instead got dismissal with a pinch of disdain. Would they keep her away from nuts? Would they use the epi-pen if she needed it? What if my daughter ate a candy bar at school, went into anaphylaxis, and died?

In the beginning, I spent a good chunk of her school time worrying that something catastrophic would happen to her. I vividly imagined getting "the call" from the school and played out tragic outcomes in my head. I imagined the emergency department scene, telling my husband what had happened, and wondered what we would say to our other child. When my own imagination couldn't conjure up enough terror, I read stories of other allergic children who had died—often at school.

What was I doing?

This indulgence in anxiety certainly wasn't good for me and it probably wasn't good for my daughter, either. By the time she got home from preschool, I was exhausted from worrying that she wouldn't come home from preschool.

Did my compulsive doom-scrolling and worrying reduce her chance of dying from an accidental nut exposure? Not at all. Action makes a difference, but worrying simply puts a pall on the day without reducing the risk, even a tiny bit, of whatever crisis you are worrying about.

Over time I became clearer about the value of action and the uselessness of worry. I taught my daughter to only eat what came from home and to self-inject her EPIPEN®. I met with teachers, cafeteria chefs, and school principals, and I presented to her class every year so her friends could learn to look out for her. I made special cupcakes that her teachers could pull from the freezer when a mom showed up unexpectedly with birthday treats. And as she got older, I took her to teen-focused food allergy conferences so she could learn how to ask a boy not to eat nuts for dinner if the date might end with a kiss.

Importantly, for my own wellbeing, I learned that after controlling everything that I could possibly control, it was best to "let go" of the outcome. What was ultimately going to happen was simply out of my control. If I got the dreaded call from the school I would deal with it then, but what was the point of imagining a catastrophe that hadn't actually happened? It is magical thinking to believe that worry would prevent her death. It wouldn't. We must also look out for the false belief that worry equals love. Did I love my daughter any less when I allowed myself to enjoy the time that she was at school? Of course not. And I was almost certainly a more relaxed and fun-loving parent when she came home than I would have been if I'd spent hours imagining her death.

Our worried brain tells us that if there is a risk, we must worry about it. It insists that we have no choice, particularly if someone we love may be in danger. If we don't worry, who knows what will happen? And what kind of person doesn't worry about their loved one who could die? What are you, a sociopath?

But this is a false belief. Worry doesn't keep anyone safe. It is actions that keep people safe. Worry is only helpful to spur action, and then it is no longer needed. I needed to be worried enough to make my daughter's special cupcakes and teach her friends how to recognize anaphylaxis. After that, my worry was harmful rather than helpful, and it was time to send it packing.

Here's the craziest thing. Not only is worry not helpful after it creates action, but the thing we choose to worry about may be entirely the wrong thing.

When I was a practicing family physician, I saw about thirty patients a day. Many people had high blood pressure or high cholesterol. Some of them had headaches or trouble sleeping. And some had a new pain or ache or fever. One busy day, I was zipping around the office and popped into an exam room to find a twelve-year-old boy, Jason, and his mom waiting to see me. We were chatty and light, everyone assuming that this would be a quick and easy visit. The mom asked how long the visit would take because she had a few more errands to run that day. She had to take the dog to the groomer, go to the garden store, and drop off the dry cleaning. There was no scary music to warn her of what was coming.

"What can I do for you today?" I asked Jason.

"My leg hurts," he said.

Had he fallen? Nope. Sports? Nope. Banged into a table? Nope. Cut his leg? Nope. He had no fever or rash or night sweats. The pain had just appeared in his left thigh about three weeks ago and had been getting steadily worse. It ached and nothing seemed to make it better. For the past few days, it had been waking him from sleep every time he rolled over.

I felt a funny feeling on the back of my neck and my chest got tight.

"Hop up here so I can take a look," I said calmly.

I had to make an intentional effort to sound light and casual because a dark dread was building inside me. He had no outward evidence of what was happening inside his leg. There was no cut or bruise or rash, and the rest of Jason's physical exam was that of a normal twelve-year-old boy. When I pushed on his left upper thigh he jumped and made a noise through clenched teeth. His mom sat calmly on a plastic chair in the corner, scrolling on her phone.

Jason's leg was thin, and I could feel his femur. Instead of a smooth, straight bone, I felt a hard, irregular, tender lump.

When I told his mom that I was concerned and we needed to get an x-ray that day, she was annoyed. She had a lot to do, and this interruption was not in her plans.

"I'm sure it's nothing," his mom said, "Can't we just wait and do it next week if he doesn't get better?"

"No." I answered firmly. "We can't."

I ordered the x-ray STAT, waited anxiously for the radiologist's report, and went back into the exam room to explain to Jason and his mom what it showed. We talked about how a bone biopsy is done and which oncologist he would go to if the biopsy was abnormal. I imagined his mom's agony when she looked up osteosarcoma that night.

The day before our visit, Jason's mom had probably worried about whether he vaped or smoked marijuana or hid vodka in his backpack. She might have worried that he wouldn't be good at sports or would be bullied at school. Maybe she worried that he'd gotten a D on a math test, didn't have many friends, or that he was mean to his sister. Maybe she worried that he would break his arm playing football. Maybe she worried that he would die in a car crash. All that worry would have been for nothing, because I'm pretty sure that she never, even for a moment, worried that he would die of cancer before he became a teenager.

While we all know we will die someday of something, we have no idea when or how. Receiving a tough diagnosis, and doom-scrolling through medical blogs, makes that illness loom large, but it doesn't change the fundamental reality that while we all die of something, the timeline and cause are a mystery.

On June 24, 2021, at a little after 1:00 a.m., The Champlain Towers South condominium in Surfside, Florida, collapsed. In the twelve seconds that it took for that oceanfront building to collapse, almost one hundred people lost their lives. I'll bet that not one of them went to bed worrying that this would be their when and how.

There were elderly couples, couples in midlife, and newlyweds. There were people in their eighties and nineties who had probably expected to die from an illness listed on their medical chart. There were young adults, teenagers, and children who were certainly not expected to die before their parents. The man in his twenties with muscular dystrophy most likely expected that his illness would contribute to his death, but it didn't. There was a Jet Blue flight attendant who might have had occasional worries about dying in a plane crash. She died in her bed.

One woman in her forties was in the condo alone because her husband was out of town on business. They were talking on the phone at 1:22 a.m. when he heard the phone line suddenly cut off. His wife had probably told him to be careful on his trip and get home safely. They couldn't have imagined that she was the one who wouldn't be safe. One terminally ill man, who lived across town, lost two sons in those towers. I'm certain that no one in that family worried more about the sons than the father. A seven-year-old little girl, whose father was a firefighter, died in the collapse. Her family must have expended much more energy worrying about her dad than about her.

One twenty-three-year-old young woman had just come to the U.S. from Paraguay. Just days before the tragedy, she had left her thatched roof home to work as a nanny for the sister of the country's First Lady. No one could have imagined that the biggest threat to this woman's life would be sleeping in a bed in a luxury Florida condo.

Okay, terrible things happen sometimes. Why do we have to think about that? you might ask.

I get it. Spending too much time thinking about tragic events gets heavy and sad and it feels much better not to think about them. Think of it like a hot stove. If we didn't feel the pain at all, we wouldn't pull our hand away and we'd get terribly burned. The pain gives us an important message, but then pulling away from the pain is protective.

What is the message from tragedies like the Surfside condo collapse? It is an invitation to put aside our magical thinking and actively live the life that is right in front of us. We do not know when we will die or how. We only know that right now we are alive and someday we won't be. That is all we need to know. Giving too much attention to guesses about how our future will play out is both useless and unhelpful. It can suck the joy out of today.

The best approach is to "control what you can and let go of the outcome." Worrying doesn't make the scary thing more or less likely to happen, but not taking appropriate action might. Drive the speed limit, get a prostate exam, take your medicines, show up for radiation, and call 911 if you get crushing chest pain. But don't spend your precious days on Earth conjuring up an imagined terrible future. What will come, will come. You'll deal with it when you have to. But if it isn't happening today, don't conjure up a sad or scary future reality. Control what you can, then let go of the outcome.

My daughters have matching black sweatshirts with huge white lettering on the back that says, "YOUR ANXIETY IS LYING TO YOU."

I love these sweatshirts.

Your anxiety *is* lying to you. It works hard to convince you that it knows the truth. It tells you that if you or someone you love is at risk of harm, the only reasonable approach is to continually imagine, in excruciating detail, all the terrible things that could happen. It tells you that you have no choice but to feel this way. It is certain that if bad things *could* happen, you are obligated to focus on them. Your anxiety is lying to you.

So, when my patient asks, "How am I supposed to live my life now that I know I'm going to die?"

The answer, of course, is, "the way you always have."

Just because your loved one has received a diagnosis doesn't mean that they will, or won't, die from their condition. They might. Or they might not. And if they do, you can't know when. Any attempt to 'figure it out' is simply magical thinking that is unhelpful. Until you, or your loved one, are at the very end of life, the path off this planet is unclear. The good news is that because it is unclear, we don't need to give our precious time and attention to this completely unanswerable question.

Control what you can and let go of the rest. Simply live your life. Not because you don't have things that you *could* worry about. I know that you do. But because worrying won't change the future, and it will ruin the present.

The state that you're shooting for is 'aware but less affected.' You understand what is going on, but once you've done all you can to control what is within your power, I want you to try to put the worry on a shelf and live the moment that you're in. Plant your garden or work on your car or make a fruit tart or watch a funny movie. When your mind goes to the scary place, gently but firmly bring it back to what you're doing right now.

I know that this is much easier for me to say than for you to do.

I also know that my patients and families who adopted this approach felt better. They felt less swallowed by fear and more in control of their day-to-day life. They weren't perfect, but they did their best. Some days were harder than others. The more they practiced the easier it got.

You will certainly have times when the fear looms large. Some days you will try to put your fear on a shelf, and it just won't stay there. That's okay. Be gentle with yourself. If you need to, you can spend a little time with the scary stuff. Sometimes it can be helpful to look the monster deep in the eyes, just don't stay there too long. If you can, after a few minutes, take some deep breaths, rub your hands together until they feel warm, and intentionally redirect your attention to your cooking or your dog or your book. You will have to do this over and over, and that's just fine. The more you practice, the easier it will get. You'll notice your fear, remind yourself that you've taken all the action that you can take, and then you'll focus your attention on something that interests you or makes you happy. You might even want to say these words out loud: "I've controlled what I can, so now I'll let go of the outcome."

Every now and then you might need to fully feel the feels. That's perfectly okay, and sometimes it can even be helpful. Releasing pent up emotion can be cleansing, like a windy day with all the doors and windows open that sweeps the dust bunnies from under the couch. The goal though, is to set some parameters around the experience so you don't get blown away. I suggest that you set a timer for fifteen minutes and let yourself rage or scream or cry. Go for the full-on ugly cry. Wail and punch the pillows, rock back and forth, and wipe your nose on your sleeve. Don't hold back. But when the timer goes off, your time is up. Bring your attention back into the room, slow your breathing, and blow your nose. Then splash some cold water on your face, take a few slow, deep breaths, and go live the day that is in front of you.

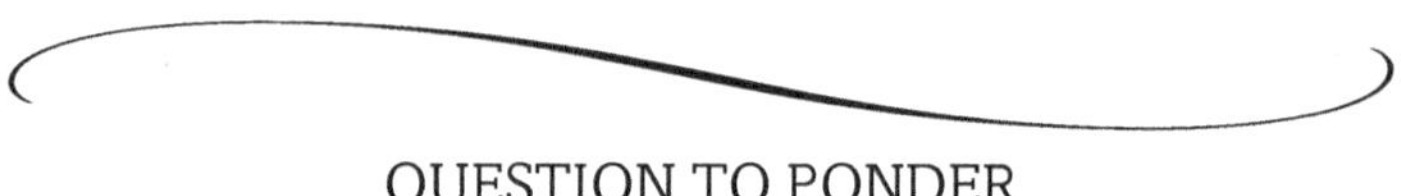

QUESTION TO PONDER

What ideas do you harbor about worrying? Do you secretly feel that worrying keeps bad things away or shows how much you care about someone?

FAMILY DISCUSSION QUESTION

What does "control what you can and let go of the rest" mean to you?

EXERCISE

Make a list of all the things that make you feel stressed. Circle the ones that you can control. These are the ones to take action on. If you catch yourself ruminating on the others, say "STOP" out loud or in your head, rub your hands together five times, take three deep breaths, and let the thought go. Repeat as often as necessary.

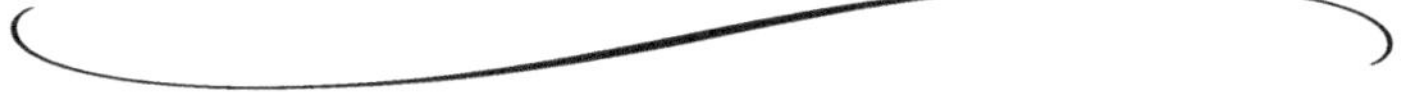

CHAPTER 8

Face the Darkness

I first met David in a patient examination room. His long body was folded into a chair that seemed too unsubstantial for the gravity of our discussion. His oncologist had sent David to me to address his cancer-related abdominal pain and his inability to sleep. I suspect that he also made the referral because David's emotional distress followed him like a cloud.

David could not accept what was happening to him.

He was consumed by the unfairness of being hit with an unstoppable illness while he was still closer to forty than fifty. It just didn't make sense, and he was certain that there must be a solution to his nightmare.

"I'm only f*cking forty-four," he blurted out in a tone louder and angrier than he meant to.

He caught himself and lowered his voice, but his agony filled the room.

"I have a son," David said. "And he's got no one other than me."

His voice got softer. "I'm forty-four, doc. It isn't fair. There has to be something you doctors can do about this."

David had stage IV colon cancer. While he had been going about his life, the cancer had silently oozed its way into his bones and his liver, threatening David's dream of seeing his son get the first academic degree in the family.

"He's in college, you know," David told me. "He's so smart. I'm proud of him, real proud. I'm going to see him graduate."

His eyes filled up. Mine filled up, too. Partly because his expansive love for his son touched me deeply, but mostly because I knew that he would not watch that beloved son walk across the graduation stage and shake hands with the dean. That talented, strong, accomplished young man would face that important day without a parent tearing up in the audience. David was right. It just wasn't fair.

We mulled over fairness for a while. And we talked about God.

"Why would God let this happen to me?" he asked, holding my gaze with piercing eyes.

I had no answer.

"I have no idea," I said. "It shouldn't be this way."

He was quiet for a long time.

"I did some bad things, doc," he said.

I knew that this was an important moment, and it was crucial not to gloss over it.

"Are you feeling like that's related to your cancer somehow?" I asked.

"Probably. Yeah. I think so," he said. "Do *you* think I'm being punished?" he asked me.

I saw the crease between his eyebrows deepen and his shoulders hunch forward. He shook his head slowly and looked at the floor.

I was tempted to jump right in with, "no, no, of course not!" but I checked myself and took a few slow, deep breaths before answering. He was taking the risk of allowing some deep spiritual pain into his awareness, and I didn't want to whitewash it and drive it back underground.

"Well . . . I don't really know how God or the Universe works," I said. "But the force that I believe in is based in love, not punishment. You may have done some bad things, but in my personal and professional opinion, bad behavior doesn't cause cancer."

"I hope you're right," he said.

We both sat in silence for a while. I fought the urge to fill up the quiet with my own voice.

"I've done some good things too," he said quietly.

"Like your son," I offered with a smile.

"Yeah," he laughed. "Like my son. He's the best thing I've ever done."

I asked if he wanted to talk to a chaplain or spiritual leader, but he wasn't interested.

"I don't need one of those. I got you, doc!" he joked.

We both laughed, and the energy in the room felt lighter.

Fear thrives in the darkness.

The idea that his cancer was punishment for past mistakes had been gnawing at David, just underneath his awareness. It made his gut feel heavy and his heart ache. The thought that his past imperfect choices were going to leave his son fatherless had been unbearable. He hadn't been aware of the burden he'd been carrying until he'd blurted it out in our meeting.

The inclination to drive our painful and frightening thoughts into the basement of our mind is powerful. We chase that snarling thought monster down the stairs and slam the door shut. Yet, even locking that door with keys and chains and padlocks won't make us feel safe, because we hear him growling and pacing under our feet. We can't see the thought monster, but we know he's still there.

There are many dark feelings that end up locked underground. My patients have locked up guilt for things they did and for things they meant to do but never got around to. They've locked up anger at God, estrangement from relatives, mean words, emotionally abandoned children, and buckets of painful emotions. Making peace with your monsters can help you shed the heaviness that makes you weary and dims your joy. No matter what you have done, who you are, or what you are facing, you deserve to be bathed in the light of acceptance and love.

When I saw David a few months later, he was angry.

"This is bullsh*t!" he yelled, pacing in the small exam room.

He was at least six foot three, maybe taller, and his agitated energy filled the room. I knew him well by now and I was concerned for him, but I wasn't afraid.

"There has to be something you doctors can do," he said loudly. "There *has* to be something."

"You seem pissed off today. What's up?" I asked.

I saw his eyes flash and his back stiffen.

"How do I know they're giving me the treatments that work?" he asked in an intense and suspicious voice.

"Tell me more about what you mean," I said.

"I'm no dummy!" he said. "I know how the world works. I'm not rich and I'm not white. How do I know I'm getting the best treatments? The ones that work. How do I know that?"

David was desperately trying to save his own life, and he was deeply concerned that he wasn't getting the best possible medical care. He worried that, because of who he was, he was being denied effective treatments that would have allowed him to live. His anger was entirely understandable given historical realities and the huge stakes that he was facing, but it created a negative feedback loop that usually ended up making him feel worse. He would get angry at his medical team, and he could sense their annoyance coming back his way. This reinforced his worry that they were holding back the best treatments that could have saved his life.

For a long time, he didn't share this concern with anyone on his treatment team, but he couldn't stop thinking about it. He knew he was getting a reputation for being an angry patient, which frustrated him because he knew himself to be a very kind and gentle person. He sensed that this anger, which bubbled up from his unexpressed fear of getting inadequate care, was making him even less likely to get the best possible treatment.

Not only did David have an unrelenting, life-threatening illness, but he was certain that a cure was being withheld from him because he wasn't white, rich, and powerful. He felt like a trapped animal frantically searching for a way to save his own life. The thought that he was being denied care because of who he was, was heavy and painful. It made a terrible situation even worse.

"Tell me more about what's on your mind," I said to David.

He shared for a long time. He shared about the times that he had felt disrespected by doctors and nurses, how he'd felt ignored in the hospital and how his family members had been mistreated. He felt certain that there was a treatment that was being withheld from him, and he felt desperate to get it so that he could be around to watch his son become a man.

His story broke my heart.

I wished that I had a way to ease David's suffering. I assumed, initially, that no amount of reassurance from me, a middle-aged white doctor, that he was getting the very best treatment available, was going to fully relieve his concerns. Yet being unable to completely remove someone's pain shouldn't stop us from trying to ease it, at least a little. Whether you are a friend, daughter, son, parent, sibling, nurse, physician, or anyone else facing another person's pain, please try not to look away.

When people have profoundly painful feelings or thoughts, such as fear of injustice, death, or retribution, you may feel so overwhelmed by the depth of their pain that you feel compelled to avert your gaze. It's this feeling of overwhelm that stops some people from donating to charities that feed hungry children or care for abandoned animals. The problem is so huge, you might think, what is the point of sending twenty dollars? But every dollar adds to every other dollar, and each one matters. Similarly, every morsel of grace, affection, or attention that you give to another person in pain matters. People need to feel seen and have their experience validated, and you always have this gift to give.

"I can't make him feel better," you might think. "I'm not a therapist or priest or rabbi or imam. What can *I* do?"

You can do a lot.

You only need to bring a tiny amount of love or light to lessen another person's suffering; you do not need to solve their whole problem. Please don't let your unrealistic desire to make a brutally hard thing magically better stop you from sharing your particular form of light.

I couldn't solve racial injustice in the U.S. healthcare system, but what I could do was validate David's perspective.

"I know that this happens," I said. "Not everyone gets treated the same in our healthcare system, so I can see why you feel the way you do. I wish you didn't need to worry about this on top of everything else that you have to worry about."

Just hearing that he didn't have to fight for, or hide, his deep worry that he was being discriminated against seemed to loosen David's heaviness just a little.

"I will look out for you," I told him. "I hear what you're saying, and I will look out for you. Here's what I know: you have excellent doctors, and you are getting the same type of treatments that I've seen other patients in your situation get, including the rich white men!"

We both laughed.

I offered to look up the expert recommended treatments for him so he could review them and make sure he was getting the best care. He sat back in the small, plastic chair, crossed his lanky legs, and smiled.

"Nah, that's okay," he said. "I guess if you're looking out for me, doc, that's good enough."

Unearthing David's dark, secret fear, shining a light on it, and validating his perspective helped him feel less at risk and less alone in the struggle. Knowing about his concern made me better able to support him as he walked his very difficult road.

When a superstar actor, who shared David's age and skin color, died of the same cancer that David had, I mentioned it at our next visit.

"You know, he could have had any treatment in the whole world," I told David. "If there were a treatment that could have cured his cancer, he would have gotten it. This cancer is just a beast."

Ironically, it was the death of this wealthy actor that most helped David come to terms with his own progressive and incurable cancer. He finally believed that there wasn't a magical treatment out there that he was being denied. He had simply been dealt a terribly sad and difficult hand.

The moral is, don't run away from the dark places. Crack open the door, shine a flashlight into the darkness, and peek inside. This won't magically make painful things happy, but it may make them just a little less heavy.

Willingness to face the darkness can strengthen relationships and make your loved one feel less afraid and less alone. Don't try to fix the unfixable. Imagine yourself walking beside the person who you love on their journey. You don't need to carry them or put their backpack of heavy junk on top of your own. It's enough to validate their experience with a simple "your backpack looks heavy," and walk beside them on the path.

Sadness is rough.

It's hard to feel sad and it's hard to watch someone that you care about be sad. If sadness is hard, depression is brutal. Knowing the difference is crucial.

When I saw Mary's name on my patient schedule, I took a slow, deep breath. I felt a heaviness even before I walked into the room.

She was deeply depressed, and she knew it. She didn't cry much, but she felt flat most of the time. Nothing made Mary happy anymore, not even her beloved little girl. She didn't care about food or sex, and although she was exhausted all day long, when it was time to sleep, she couldn't.

She had tried an antidepressant once, but she hated the way it made her feel. She'd sworn off antidepressants for good, and I could not get her to reconsider.

"Every medication is different," I told her. "Just because you had a weird reaction to one medicine doesn't mean another antidepressant would affect you in the same way."

She was unmoved.

"I am never taking one of those things again. No way," she told me.

This decision was reducing her quality of life, I thought, and that made me sad. I tried to reach her through logic, by explaining that I could choose a medication with a completely different mechanism of action. I tried to reach her through emotion by highlighting how much better it would be for her young daughter if her mommy weren't so depressed. I tried a compromise by offering a reduced dose, slow titration, or an herbal treatment rather than a pharmaceutical. Nope. She wasn't interested.

Ultimately, I simply accepted that Mary had the right to make decisions for her health that she felt good about, and it wasn't my place to bully her into choosing what I thought she should do. We explored many non-medication approaches to treating her depression, including acupuncture, meditation, yoga, exercise, and journaling. I was thrilled when she finally agreed to see a therapist for cognitive behavioral therapy. Over time, the gray film that had covered everything in Mary's life, dampening her joy, started to lift. She laughed more, felt more hopeful, and her sleep returned. I feel fairly certain that an antidepressant would have relieved her suffering faster, but I was happy that Mary had found a plan that worked for her.

Depression sucks. It sucks the enjoyment out of life, makes easy things hard and hard things nearly impossible.

People who are depressed don't always seek treatment, but it would almost always be better if they did. There are many tools to help relieve depression. There are medications of course, such as SSRIs (selective serotonin reuptake inhibitors) and SNRIs (serotonin and norepinephrine reuptake inhibitors), and for some people these can be life changing. It isn't a personal failure to take antidepressants any more than it is to take blood pressure medicines if you have hypertension or insulin if you have diabetes. Depression is a life-threatening, happiness reducing illness, and if you have it, you deserve to feel better. Depression is treatable, and if a healthcare expert who you trust has suggested that you consider antidepressants, please take a breath, calm your initial resistance, and consider if following their advice might make your life a little better. If you have a whispered, secret feeling after reading this paragraph that I might be talking to you, please call your doctor and ask them to assess you for depression. If you do that, end up getting treated for depression, and then feel better, please email me and tell me about it. You'll make my day!

There are many treatments for depression other than medications, and a combination of treatments usually works better than one method alone. Therapy is wonderful, and if you are reading this book, you should probably consider finding a great therapist. Having serious illness in the family, whether in your body or the body of someone that you love, is destabilizing, terrifying, and exhausting. It helps to process this with another person who can teach you skills that will significantly improve your coping. Cognitive Behavioral Therapy (CBT) and Mindfulness Based Cognitive Therapy (MBCT) are two techniques that can fundamentally improve your wellbeing. Mindfulness Based Stress Reduction (MBSR) is another useful tool. Look it up—you'll be impressed. It is a fantastic research-proven program that reduces depression, anxiety, pain, sleep problems, stress, and more. Once you learn the techniques, you can do them in your own home, all by yourself. Other proven options for treating depression include acupuncture, exercise, and yoga. There are also more aggressive approaches like Transcranial Magnetic Stimulation and ketamine that you can chat with your doctor about if other methods haven't helped.

If you're depressed, I would like you to actively pursue treatment to be less depressed. You deserve to feel better. The voice in your head that says "it won't work, anyway" is the depression talking and he is a big, nasty liar; don't believe a word he says. Also, depression shows up differently in different people. Not everyone who is depressed cries, and plenty of people who cry are not depressed. When depression sneaks in, it is like wearing sunglasses inside. Everything just feels dim. Things that used to matter feel flat or irrelevant or impossible or blah. The movie view of the weeping, depressed woman is cliché, and while clichés usually have a kernel of truth, they never tell the whole story. Depression tends to make people isolate, and it takes the color out of the world. It messes up sleep, appetite, and concentration, and it can make you feel guilty even when you have nothing to feel guilty about. In some people, typically men, but not exclusively of course, depression can show up as crankiness or anger.

"Have you been more irritable lately?" I've asked many men who I suspected of being depressed.

They often say "no," and then I look to the spouse who has eyes as wide as bottle caps and is frantically nodding their head up and down.

One of depression's most powerful tricks is called anhedonia. Anhedonia means that things that you enjoyed in the past have somehow lost their juice. You don't care about reading the newspaper anymore or knitting or woodworking or online shopping. You back out of family activities, and even your adorable chihuahua doesn't make you smile anymore. Of course, being seriously ill can make you feel lousy, which can suck the fun out of activities, too. However, if a letter from your beloved granddaughter doesn't make you smile, you might have anhedonia.

Sometimes, the darkness gets so thick that you can no longer imagine the light. This is a dangerous time that sometimes leads a person to take their own life. If you are feeling this way right now, please put this book down and call someone immediately. You can ask a friend to take you to the emergency department, call 911, or call a suicide hotline. Suicide is a permanent decision. There are no do overs. Depression can be temporary, but suicide is forever. I don't want this to happen to you. You matter on this Earth, and you can absolutely feel better with help. I am 100 percent certain that you can enjoy life again and get your old self back. If you feel seen after reading this paragraph, like I somehow crawled into your head and read your mind, go call someone right now. Please.

If you're still reading, I'm going to assume that you're safe.

Depression isn't sadness and sadness isn't depression, but they often hang out together.

Not everyone who is bummed out is depressed. Sadness is a normal emotion that tends to accompany loss. The loss might be a person or a beloved pet or a home or job or possession. Sadness may also follow a loss of a body part (such as a breast), a dream (such as having a baby), or a fervent hope (such as a cure for a serious illness). Sadness isn't fun, but it is a part of being human.

Sadness doesn't require treatment. It is part of the human experience, and sometimes the right approach is just to feel it. You might let your sadness wash over you and touch your deepest, softest parts. On some level, sadness is an expression of love. If you didn't care, the loss wouldn't hurt. Tears can be a balm or a rinsing away of layers of emotional crud. They can leave you exposed and raw, yet open to renewal and connection. Sadness has healing potential.

Also, sadness is a drag. It is exhausting and a bummer, and you might have had enough of it. If you're tired of the whole "healing tears" idea, you might be interested in some tools for managing your sadness. There's no pill to treat it, but there are things that can help.

Share It

Often, sadness is heavier when you bear it alone. If you're lost in the dark it can feel comforting to have someone walking beside you, even if neither of you has any idea where you're going. Whether you're the kind of person who finds comfort in handling tough things alone, or one who finds strength in connection, sharing your sadness can help. You don't need to have an empathetic best friend or a fabulously caring spouse. If you do, good for you. But if you don't, that's fine too. You can share with your dog or cat or bearded dragon. You can talk to yourself in the shower. You can talk to someone on the TV, in an online support group, or you can write in a journal. You can have a whole conversation with yourself while you clean the house. It doesn't matter how you share your sadness, just don't keep it locked up inside your head or your heart.

Accept It

Fighting against sadness pumps it up. Acceptance doesn't mean you like something, or you don't wish it were different. Of course you wish it were different. But there is a tightness to trying to hold off sadness. Imagine that sadness is trying to bust through the door and you're using all your energy to keep the door shut. While you've got your shoulder against the door and your feet dug into the ground, you can't be dancing or snuggling or calmly enjoying the cicada song in the back yard. Fighting against sadness steals energy for much more enjoyable pursuits. What if you back away from the door and allow sadness to come in and plop onto the couch? He'll be there, and he'll probably be annoying. But while he annoys you quietly from the living room, you can be cooking or drawing or laughing with a friend. Sadness is there, but it doesn't have to be all about him.

Create Rituals

There is a reason that many cultures have rituals surrounding the ultimate sadness that accompanies the loss of a loved one. They help.

Yet funerals and memorial services don't have to be the only rituals in our toolbox. When my beloved poodle died, I made an art piece with his fuzzy face in it. I cried while I worked on it, but it helped. I remembered his goofy times, his cuddly times, and my tears had an "I love you" vibe to them. There was a sweetness there.

On the first anniversary of my daughter's horse accident, we made a cake that said "F*ck last year." She was starting to feel a little better, but we weren't ready to just be grateful and move on quite yet. We wanted to mark how tough and crappy the past year had been. The cake was delicious, and we felt a weird sort of power as we ate it. We had survived the worst of the storm and it felt good to give an F-you to all the pain and fear and uncertainty of the year before.

What creative rituals might help you? Here are some ideas:

I love you rituals: There are so many ways to express love. You could make an art piece, a collage, a journal, a crocheted blanket, or a song. You could plant a tree or create a memorial corner with pictures and mementos. You could incorporate poems or prayers or a meditation over coffee. Try brainstorming a whole page of ideas, from practical ones to silly and outside-the-box options. Read your list the next day and find a few I love you rituals that resonate.

F-you rituals: The F-you cake is a personal favorite, but certainly not the only option. You could write down the things that you are sad about and rip the paper into shreds or burn it in the fireplace. You could write an F-you poem or draw your sadness like an ugly monster. You could have an F-you party and take turns yelling at whatever is making you sad.

Give back rituals: Turning your attention to helping other people can allow a little light into the dark places. You could make blankets for women with ovarian cancer getting chemotherapy. Or snuggle lonely shelter dogs. You could write letters of support to overseas soldiers or play cards with hospice patients. The giving back may be related to what your family is struggling with, but it certainly doesn't have to be. Sadness is self-focused, so sometimes any other-focused action can lighten the heaviness just a little.

Let it go rituals: When the time is right, letting go of the sadness that things haven't turned out as you'd hoped can be powerfully healing. It makes space for whatever the next phase is going to be. There are endless ways to create a 'let it go' ritual, including scattering seeds, creating a small memorial out of leaves and sticks and sending it down a stream, prayers sent skyward, and scattering ashes. Writing in a journal, drumming, "blowing away" pain with the breath, and whole-body shaking are other ways to let go of painful emotions that feel stuck.

Perhaps the most important concept to understand when thinking about sadness is "the only way out is through." You can spend an enormous amount of energy fighting your sadness, running away from it, or trying to stuff it into the basement and pretending it isn't there. If that worked, I'd be all for it. Unfortunately, it doesn't. Pushing away your painful feelings when they are asking to be acknowledged doesn't eliminate them, but it does take a tremendous amount of energy just when your reserves are low.

What if you tried this approach instead? Gather your courage, straighten your spine, puff out your chest, take a few deep breaths, open the door, and let those feelings in. This way, you decide when the door gets opened and you don't have to work so brutally hard to keep it closed. The feelings won't unexpectedly burst in during an important meeting, and you'll have more energy to put towards your own healing.

Ironically, the more you welcome the waves of sadness, share your experience with your tribe, and create rituals to help you move forward, the more quicky you will get to the other side.

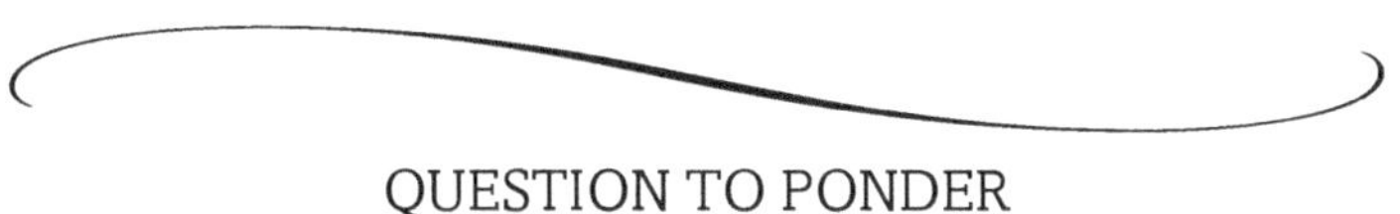

QUESTION TO PONDER

Are there any strong feelings, fears, or sadness that you have locked in your 'basement?'

FAMILY DISCUSSION QUESTION

Are the members of our family suffering with sadness, depression, or both?

EXERCISE

Choose a ritual to help process your sadness and practice it this week.

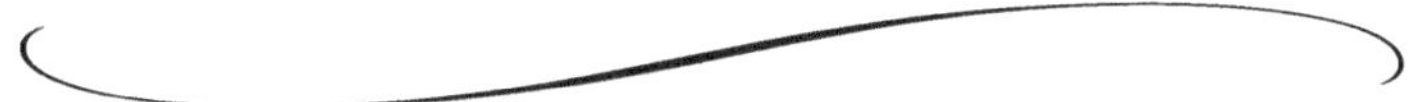

CHAPTER 9

Focus on the Now

Amanda worried too much.

A forty-six-year-old woman with a full-time professional career and four children, Amanda led a busy life. She was financially comfortable and had created the life she had always thought she would want, but she couldn't seem to relax, even when there were no immediate crises with her work or her family. Amanda often felt on edge.

"I don't know what's wrong with me," she told me. "I know nothing is wrong, but I still always *feel* like something is wrong."

I asked about her support system, and she said, "My husband is my biggest supporter, I guess. But he's away on business so much that I'm basically a single parent."

I asked Amanda about her kids.

"They're a mess," she said at first. Then she qualified her answer. "No, not really. They're great. But they worry all the time, and they have a lot going on. It's hard to be a kid, you know?"

I nodded.

"I think we're all kind of a mess," she said. "When one of us gets overwhelmed or riled up, the whole family falls apart."

"What are some of the biggest stressors in your life right now?" I asked Amanda.

I knew that Amanda had had breast cancer in her late thirties, and she shared that she had a nagging, low grade worry that it would come back. She couldn't shake the feeling that disaster was about to strike.

"Every time I feel tired or have a pain or a cough, I'm sure that that's it for me," she said. "It feels like some catastrophe is about to hit me and I need to prepare myself."

"I worry about my kids all the time," Amanda said. "What if they don't have good friends, or get a spot on their sports team, or a part in the play? I even worry that my worrying will mess them up," she said, and we both laughed.

Amanda shared that she knew she had good kids and she trusted them to make good decisions, but she also knew that life could throw you a curve ball at any time and she wanted to be prepared. Even though there was a lot in her life for which she felt grateful, it just didn't feel safe to Amanda to simply relax and enjoy her life.

"What else feels stressful?" I asked.

"I worry about my dad a lot," Amanda shared. "He's eighty-two and he lives alone, and he's starting to seem . . . I don't know . . . old," she said. "He's always been so independent and strong, and he's kind of the rock of the family. I never really thought he'd get old."

Amanda smiled when she talked about her dad. Her obvious love for him was heartwarming.

"We used to have such a close relationship," she said, "but now he always seems annoyed with me. He doesn't understand that at his age he needs to eat better, stop watching so much TV, and stop smoking. He needs to do brain games every day and has got to stop eating sweets."

I was starting to understand why Amanda's dad was feeling annoyed.

"I just don't want him to die," she said. "I couldn't handle that. That's why he has to take care of himself. God, he's so stubborn. If he would just take better care of himself, I could relax."

The more we talked, the more I understood how pervasive Amanda's anxiety was. She worried about all the things, all the time. She worried that her boss wasn't happy with her, that her coworkers didn't really like her, that her house wasn't decorated well enough, and that her neighbors were judging her dog's poor behavior. She worried about her eating habits, her weight, her clothes, her messy closets, and her future.

If Amanda could think about it, she could worry about it.

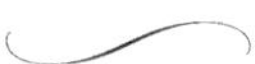

Amanda's worry was sucking the joy out of her life.

Our long-ago ancestors, the early humans who came before us, lived with constant physical threat. Food wasn't assured, hungry predators prowled around looking to fill their bellies, and there were no door locks or house alarms to keep other people away from our ancestors' stuff. Despite this rough life, it is likely that some early humans tended more toward the "I'm sure it's fine" point of view, while others imagined disaster around every corner. In this harsh environment, being too chill and missing the lion hiding in the grass could have created a survival disadvantage. The "Oh no, we're in trouble" people might have kept themselves safer, and therefore lived longer, while the "don't worry about it" folks might have ended up as lion chow. Assuming that noises in the night or rustles in the grass were friendly visitors might have meant a shorter life and fewer babies.

Our ancestors were likely to be worriers.

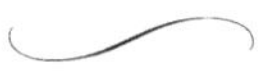

Just like a little salt makes a dish taste better but too much makes it inedible, a little worry helps keep us safe, but too much ruins our experience of living.

Here's the thing about worry: most of the things that you worry about could actually happen. You could lose your job, your dog, or your loved one. People could talk about you behind your back or steal the candy bars from your desk drawer. That dress might, in fact, make your butt look big.

Because our anxiety helped us avoid becoming a lion snack way back when, it now thinks that it has the right to beat us over the head with all the things in our life that could go wrong. And we can't even be mad about it because there really is no shortage of terrible things that *could* happen—car crashes, breakups, pandemics, house fires, oozing skin rashes, dogs with bloody diarrhea, or kids who bring home a fiancé with offensive body odor. My active imagination could fill a notebook with potential tragedies, and I'll bet that yours could too.

So, when someone says, "Don't worry," our natural instinct is to fight back. "Why shouldn't I worry? Let me tell you about all the awful things that could happen to me and the people that I love."

This tendency to catastrophize, imagining all the terrible things that could happen, started as a protective approach and for many people it is simply part of who they are. We need these people though, because they are the ones who take your car keys when you've had too much to drink or double-check that the candles were blown out before you leave the house to go to the movies.

But here's the key: we get to decide where we put our attention.

Right now, at this very moment, one of my children could die in a car crash or be pushed off a subway platform. My husband could have a heart attack or my chihuahua, with her collapsing trachea, could asphyxiate right in front of my eyes. Yikes! Just writing that made my pulse speed up and my chest feel tight. Those things are all possible, but I actively choose not to pay attention to those possibilities.

Instead, I've decided to pay attention to the bird cacophony and vibrant spring plants blooming outside my window. I notice the textures in the room I'm sitting in, the strong, brown wood sculptures and the fuzzy blankets on my couch. I notice the feeling of the chair under my rear end and the slight ache of my hips from sitting too long.

I hear the whir of the air cleaners. I take a deep breath and notice the rise of my chest and the expansion of my belly. I focus on the sound of the air passing my lips as I exhale. I can feel my pulse slowing, my chest opening, and my muscles relaxing.

Nothing has changed.

That is, nothing has changed except for my attention. The key here is that we always have the choice of where we place our attention. So, when someone says "don't worry," don't hear that as "you have nothing to worry about." Instead, try to hear that direction as "may I kindly suggest that you thoughtfully choose where you want to put your attention?"

Choosing Where to Put Your Attention: Past-**Now**-Future

At any given moment, our mind can only be paying attention to one of three possibilities: things that happened in the past, things that could happen in the future, and whatever is happening right now, at this very moment. If we don't intentionally choose where to put that attention, our untrained, unhinged monkey mind will choose for us. I don't generally trust his choices.

The Unchangeable Past

Ruminating on happy things in the past is great. If that's where your monkey mind takes you, lucky you. You have a good monkey, and he deserves a banana. But if you're like the rest of us, that's not where your monkey mind usually goes. Our uncontrolled monkey minds may rummage through every past failure, shame, and sadness. They remember every time we were excluded or rejected or treated unfairly. They remind us that we used to be more vibrant, less wrinkly, and able to fit into our skinny jeans, but instead of remembering those times fondly, they beat us up for how we've declined.

This rumination about past slights and failures does nothing to improve your life. The past is over, and you can't change it, so spending any time marinating in the soup of disappointment is an exercise certain to reduce your well-being without offering any benefit. Just stop doing it.

The only exception is grieving. Grieving the loss of a person, pet, job, relationship, breast, uterus, prostate, leg, or anything else that is precious to you is healthy and normal. As part of the grieving process, you may spend time remembering how things used to be and comparing them to now. This can be hard and sad, but it is simply part of normal grieving.

Other than grieving and celebrating happy memories, and perhaps work that you are doing with a licensed therapist, don't spend much time mucking around in past failures or disappointments.

The Imaginary Future

When your monkey mind isn't cataloguing all the ways that you've failed or been wronged in the past, it is most likely telling you all the terrifying things that could happen in the future.

"Dad could fall, you know, if you don't spend every weekend with him."

"If you eat sugar your cancer will come back."

"You'll probably have terrible side effects from chemo."

The monkey could be right, of course. Dad might fall, your cancer might come back, and you might feel tired and nauseous from chemotherapy. Or the monkey could be wrong. That's the important point: just because the monkey *could* be right, doesn't mean he *will* be right. Spending time in the future worrying about things that may or may not happen is an exercise in unnecessary self-flagellation. It doesn't prevent the future bad mojo, but it does ruin today.

We need to spend a moment discussing magical thinking.

When I teach these ideas in seminars or courses, I often get at least one person who says something like, "But I worry about things so they *won't* happen."

I understand the impulse to believe that worrying keeps us safe. It would be nice if worrying were an amulet that could keep all the bad and scary things away. Unfortunately, while there are things that we can do to help keep us safe, the worrying itself doesn't do a darn thing. Worrying about Dad falling won't stop him from falling, but you know what will? Removing the throw rugs and moving the lamp cords. That will definitely help keep Dad from falling. So, you need the worry just for a moment, just long enough to remind you to move the throw rugs, and not a moment more.

If you aren't supposed to ruminate about the past or worry about the future, where are you supposed to put your attention? I would like you to focus your attention firmly in the present moment, the literal moment that you're living in right now. There is magic in the Now.

The Now

Unless someone is actively trying to kill you right this moment, the Now is generally not that bad. You are probably reasonably well fed, protected from the elements, and safe from predators. Focusing on the Now has great benefits and is one of the most powerful approaches for minimizing anxiety.

Let's practice. Take a moment to notice the moment that you are living in, right now. What do you see? Look around and notice the colors and textures around you. Try to pay attention to what you're seeing even more intensely than you normally do. Maybe you can see color variations or shadows that you've never noticed. If there is another person in the room with you, notice their eyebrows. Is the color uniform? What direction do the hairs follow? Any stragglers begging to be plucked?

Focusing on discrete parts of a person's face is a powerful technique for being present when you're with someone. It might seem odd at first, but it helps connect you to the person and stop your monkey mind from flitting around and thinking about chores or TV shows or lunch plans.

Notice what you hear. Maybe there are birds or other nature sounds, maybe you hear the sound of the dishwasher or air cleaners. Is there traffic noise? Try to tap into the sounds that normally recede out of your awareness.

Notice what you feel. Can you feel the seat under your bottom or your feet on the floor? Take one hand and run it gently over the other palm. Notice all those sensations.

Notice what you smell. Whether the smell is closer to a bouquet of flowers or a wet Newfoundland dog, simply notice it.

If you have food nearby, put a small piece in your mouth and spend some time noticing all the tastes and textures associated with that food. How does it feel on your tongue? Is it sweet or salty? Hard or mushy? Pointy or smooth?

Your five senses are always with you, and you can call on them any time you need to corral your monkey mind and bring your attention to the Now.

Noticing Your Mind

Once you start watching your mind, I predict that you'll be blown away by how much time you spend ruminating about the past or worrying about the future.

"Can you believe she treated you that way at the picnic?" your mind might ask.

Or, "I won't know anyone at the party, I'll probably have a terrible time."

Most of us bounce back and forth between the past and the future, spending an absurdly small amount of time in the moment that we're actually living.

If you're out on a walk and see a pretty flowering bush, your mind might say, "We used to have bushes like that, but they all died," or,

"The flowers came early this year, my allergies will probably be terrible this season."

If you were focusing on the Now you might simply say to yourself, "What a vibrant and beautiful pink color."

Your first task is just to notice what your mind is doing. Imagine that you are the grownup observing a clever but naughty child. "Look at what my mind is doing now," you might say to yourself. "It has dredged up some old funky memories of people being mean to me and made up that mom's new doctor probably won't be very good."

Of course, you can't spend all day, every day, focusing on your own mind because you'll drive yourself nuts and your laundry will never get done. The key is to do it when you're feeling a strong emotion. So, if you start to feel sad or agitated or angry or stressed, it is likely that your monkey mind has taken you away from the Now. That is a key time to check in with what your mind has been up to and gently redirect it back to where you want it to be.

Commanding Your Mind

You are the grown up and you get to be in charge. Once you start paying attention to what your monkey mind is doing you get to decide if you approve, or if he needs a visit to the timeout chair.

Imagine that your mind starts saying something like, "The biopsy will probably be positive. I just can't deal with that. I know the doctors will suggest chemo and I'll probably get all the side effects just like my sister did. I can't deal with losing my hair. I just can't. John will probably leave me if I'm bald. And how will we tell the kids?"

Do you have cancer? I have no idea. And will you need chemo and lose your hair? I don't know. They key, however, is that you don't know either. When you get the news, you'll know and that will be your Now. You will deal with whatever hand you're dealt. Right now, however, when your mind took you way into the future, no one on Earth knows whether or not your biopsy will be positive or if John would leave you if you're bald. So, it is not a good idea let your mind go to its imaginary playroom and scare the pants off you by telling you things that may or may not be true.

Once you notice what your mind is doing, it is up to you to take charge. When you notice it sliding down the slippery slope of "what if . . ." or "can you believe . . . ," that's your cue to step in.

One of my favorite techniques to take command of your mind is called Thought Stopping. When you notice your mind drifting to an unhelpful place, simply say "STOP," and put your hand out in front of you like a cranky school crossing guard. Then rub your hands together, until they get warm, and take a few deep breaths. This gets your monkey mind's attention.

Once you've interrupted the monkey you can intentionally choose where to focus your mind. You could notice what you see, hear, feel, smell, and taste, or you could focus on a few things that you're grateful for. You could throw a ball for your dog and pay attention to his goofy grin, or you could get carried away by a compelling book or movie. You could delve into a craft or woodworking project or focus all your attention on cleaning out a closet. You could paint your nails or create a hearty meal. You could take a hot shower. The key is to focus all your attention on whatever you are actually doing in this one moment of your one precious life.

Don't be surprised if three minutes into your project, movie, or shower your monkey mind acts up again. Expect it. It will definitely happen. Don't get mad or frustrated or give up. Just redirect your mind to your project, movie, or shower. Then do it again. And again. And again.

The more you practice this the easier it gets, and the more control you will have over your mind and your attention. With practice, you will catch your monkey mind the moment he starts slipping into rumination or worry and you'll quickly redirect him to focus on the Now.

When You Don't Like the Present Moment

I was teaching a class of medical students about these concepts and one student just wasn't having it.

"What if the present moment sucks?" he asked with a smirk. "Like what if I'm studying for a test and I hate it. Why would I want to focus on that?"

"You're exactly right," I told him. "Sometimes the present moment is tough. You could be studying or having an argument with someone special or even crying over something that happened to you. There is no guarantee that the present moment will be all sunshine and unicorns."

I paused.

"The present moment, the Now, simply *is*," I said. "It could be pleasurable, or it could be a drag. But whatever it is, it is better than ruminating about past mistakes and hurts or worrying about imaginary things that may or may not happen."

"If you're studying," I continued, "your Now is to read your notes and try to memorize them. That is helpful to you. Here's what wouldn't be helpful: agonizing that you didn't start studying earlier (the unchangeable past) or telling yourself that you're probably going to fail the exam no matter how much you study (the imaginary future)."

So, if you're studying, study. If you're crying, cry. Don't bring back into your awareness all the other times that people have made you cry or imagine that you'll never stop crying. Just cry today's tears until they're gone, then go wash your face and have some chocolate.

Not every moment in life is glorious or happy. Sometimes the Now is boring or gross or hard or sad. You may have picked up an unspoken societal message that you should run away from those moments in the relentless pursuit of joy. That is an unhelpful and unrealistic suggestion, and I hope that you'll reject it. Instead, I'd love for you to try to live fully into all the moments of your life. Some will be bitter and some will be sweet, but they are all important components of your time here on Earth. Severely traumatic experiences are one clear exception, but other than that, our moments are all precious.

Let's not waste them.

"Oh my God," Amanda said the next time I saw her. "I can't believe how crazy my monkey mind is. He's totally out of control."

We laughed.

"He doesn't take me to the past too much, but he cannot stop going to the future and telling me all of the terrible things that are going to happen to me and everyone that I care about."

"Were you able to get any control over him?" I asked her.

"Yes. I really did. Once I started noticing what he was up to I did what you said and yelled STOP and it really worked," Amanda said. "Sometimes I had to say it in my head though," she laughed, "because he acts up in public, too."

I wasn't surprised that this technique worked for Amanda because it has worked for so many of my other patients, and it also works for me. Noticing where your monkey mind is putting his attention, using thought stopping to interrupt it, and then redirecting your attention to the Now is one of the most powerful techniques for reducing worry and anxiety.

The more you practice this, the easier it will get.

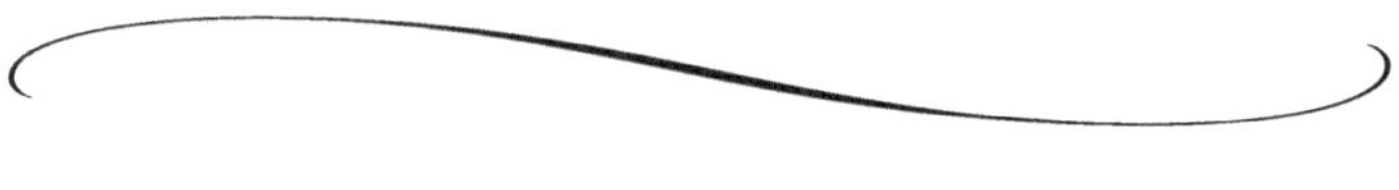

QUESTION TO PONDER

Does your monkey mind tend to spend more time ruminating about the unchangeable past or worrying about the imaginary future?

FAMILY DISCUSSION QUESTION

How could we gently remind each other to focus on the Now when our monkey minds take us to the unchangeable past or imaginary future?

EXERCISE

Write *Past-NOW-Future* on sticky notes and put them around your house to remind you to notice and redirect your mind to the Now.

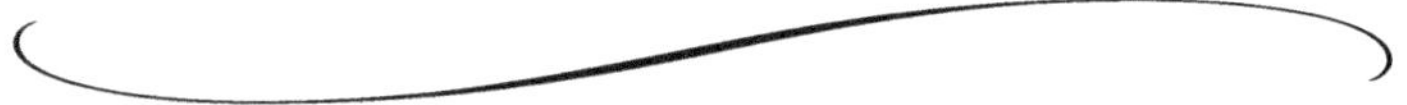

CHAPTER 10

Use the Contentment Equation

Carolina was fifty-two and overwhelmed. Her father, Andrew, was declining and her teenage son was driving her crazy. Her head hurt all day long and she was exhausted, but she couldn't even imagine another way to go through life. She felt trapped.

Her dad lived in an assisted living facility. It had been a struggle to get him there, and in the process their relationship had taken a hit. He felt like she had disrespected him and overrode his wishes to stay in his home, and she felt like he had been unrealistic about his ability to take care of himself in that huge, old, two-story house. She had hoped that once she got him to his new apartment, with staff to keep an eye on him, things would get easier. They hadn't.

Now that he'd been in his new apartment for almost a year, the shock of the move had worn off. But rather than settling into a new, positive routine, Andrew spent his time cataloging all the things that he hated about his new place. The food was disgusting, the people were snobby or dumb, and the apartment was too small. He was bored and unhappy and he made sure that Carolina knew it.

"I don't know what you want from me, Dad," Carolina said through gritted teeth. "I can't fix it, okay. I can't. There's nothing that I can do and there's no way to make you happy. I give up. I just give up."

"You can get me out of here, that's what you can do," her dad snapped back. "I wouldn't let my dog suffer like this."

Carolina felt hopeless.

Every attempt to make Andrew happy or more engaged with his new life seemed to make him more resistant and crankier. Whenever Carolina saw his name pop up on her phone, her jaw clenched, and her chest felt tight. He was making her crazy. She was pretty sure that if he got more involved in the activities at his new facility, he'd be happier, and she'd be happier. But no matter how many times she told him to do this, nothing ever changed.

Carolina was white-knuckling her way through life, but she wasn't happy. Even though she was exhausted all the time, she felt wide awake as soon as she got into bed. Her shoulders ached and her gut felt sluggish. She didn't laugh very often, and she rarely had fun.

Even when she wasn't dealing with her dad, life felt hard. Her job was stressful, her coworkers were annoying, and her son was surly and obnoxious. Carolina constantly felt like she was on the verge of a breakdown, but she knew she'd never let herself fall apart. She was the one who kept everything together. She was often angry at the people in her life because they didn't help her, but they still expected her to help them. Her son did nothing around the house but still expected his laundry done. Her husband retreated to his TV shows as soon as he got home from work, but still expected her to make dinner.

If anyone had asked Carolina how she was doing, she would have answered, "I'm a mess and life is unfair."

No one asked.

Clearly, Carolina is unhappy.

Her life is filled with negative emotions, and her mood, her body, her sleep, and her sense of the world as a joyful place have all taken a hit. She can't magically make her father younger or happier, turn her teenage son into a neat and pleasant person, or transform her indifferent husband into an adoring and supportive one.

So, is Carolina stuck, doomed to live the rest of her life as a frustrated, seething, exhausted person?

No.

Carolina is not doomed because, although she can't control what happens to her, she *can* control something very important. She can control how she responds.

There is great power in intentionally choosing your responses to negative situations and negative people. This is where your deeply impactful ability to manage your own well-being lies. When a doctor doesn't return your calls, your car breaks down on the way to a meeting, or your friend blows you off, the level of your unhappiness is impacted both by the outside forces and by what happens inside of you.

It is the combination of the unpleasantness of the experience, with the level of negativity that you add to the mix, that determines how lousy you feel.

You might even think of it like an equation.

The Contentment Equation

What You Are Facing X How You Respond =
How Satisfied/Happy/Content You Feel

Or put more simply:

Experience X Response = Contentment

This equation illustrates the magnitude of our power to control our own wellbeing by taking control of our response to challenging situations.

Rating Experiences

Just for fun, let's assign numbers to a few experiences to see how it works. Some experiences are intrinsically more positive than others, so they would have higher numbers. Lousy experiences get lower numbers. You and I might rate specific experiences differently, but the equation still works. Using a one (bad) to ten (great) scale, here's my rating of a few experiences:

- Being yelled at by a declining, cranky relative = two

- Gastrointestinal virus = three

- First bite of a delicious chocolate cake = eight

- Family travel to an awe-inspiring place = ten

The thing about experiences, particularly the tougher ones, is that you don't usually have control over if, and when, they happen. Generally, if you *can* avoid negative experiences that's what you do. Has anyone ever intentionally sought out a stomach virus? This means that if you're facing a tough experience, you probably couldn't find a way to escape it.

The Response side of the equation is different. This is where your power lies. While you can't always choose your experiences, you do have the power to choose your responses. Some people find it intrinsically easy to generate a neutral or positive response to problems, while for other people negativity rushes in at the first sign of trouble. Just as each of us has a different level of physical fitness, we each have differing abilities to bring a neutral or positive response to a challenging situation.

The good news is that this is a muscle that you can build. If you don't naturally lean towards the positive, don't worry about it. The more you practice, the better you'll get.

Rating Responses

For the purpose of the Contentment Equation, we can rate our responses numerically, like we rated our experiences. If something unpleasant happens, how might you respond? Low numbers represent a negative response and higher numbers are the more positive responses that we're shooting for. Using a one (strongly negative) to ten (strongly positive) scale, here's my rating of a few possible responses to an unpleasant experience:

Scream/smash dishes to the floor = two

Raise your voice/say mean words/feel guilty = three

Shut down/feel sorry for yourself = four

Take a deep breath/go for a short walk = seven

Use your five senses to focus on the moment and look for the gift or opportunity in the experience = nine

Let's see if it works.

Experience X Response = Contentment

Cranky relative (two) X Yell mean words/feel guilty (three) =
Low Contentment (six)

Cranky relative (two) X Take deep breaths/go for walk (seven) =
Higher Contentment (fourteen)

This is an absurd oversimplification of course, because none of our problems or strengths can be reduced to a simple number. Even if they could, we would never agree on which number to assign to which problem. For me, a yelling relative is a lousy level two, but dog diarrhea is a no-big-deal level five. If you come from a family of yelling dog haters, you might think my numbers should be reversed. So, it's more the concept than the specifics that I'd like you to ponder. The key idea is that you can't always control your experiences, but you can always, theoretically, control your response.

"But how?" you might ask. "How am I supposed to control my response when I get yelled at or pooped on or disappointed or frustrated or when the darn dishes are *still* in the sink when I get home from work?"

Your Body Tells the Story

When you're at your most Zen, annoying experiences are easier to cope with. You can laugh off other people's mistakes and put daily annoyances in perspective. A calm nervous system allows you to respond to tough experiences with neutral or positive energy.

On the other hand, an agitated nervous system, one that is stuck in the stress response, is more likely to perceive negative experiences as catastrophes. If you're in this state, a flat tire or rush hour traffic or harsh word from someone you care about can feel like the end of the world. If your body is ramped up and stressed, it is tough to respond with neutrality and calm.

The goal is to notice if your body is agitated and stressed so you can activate your nervous system-calming plan. Your body will tell the story.

When your stress response is activated, you may feel some of the following symptoms:

- Fast heart rate
- Rapid breathing
- Chest tightness
- Clenched jaw
- Headache
- Neck pain
- Hunched shoulders
- Stomach pain
- Diarrhea
- Pelvic pain
- Trouble concentrating
- Clenched fists

Your body is a strong communicator, and it will tell you when it is feeling agitated.

Not everyone responds this way, however. Some people experience a "freeze" response, or "shut down" when they feel threatened or stressed. If this sounds more like you, facing a difficult situation may result in:

- Withdrawing from people
- Spacing out
- Trouble concentrating
- Sudden and extreme fatigue

The specific response to stress that you experience isn't that important; however, it's extremely important for you to get to know yourself. What happens when you feel stressed? Do you clench your teeth, get a crampy belly, or hike your shoulders to your ears? Do you space out and become hard to reach? When I'm stressed, I tend to feel a tightness in my chest. The value of paying attention to your body in this way is that it can clue you in to escalating stress even before your conscious mind is aware of what is happening.

Take a moment now to identify where *your* body feels its stress.

When you learn to tap into your body and notice when your stress response is escalating, it gives you the power to take action *before* you send that snarky email or lash out at your annoying family member.

This is what can happen if you don't pay attention:

Annoying experience ---> Agitated response ---> Unpleasant consequences

This approach is better:

Annoying experience ---> Notice your body's response ---> Calming practice ---> Neutral outcome

Let's look at a more practical example:

Your brother criticizes you ---> You yell at him ---> He storms out ---> Everyone feels badly

Or:

Your brother criticizes you ---> You notice that your jaw is clenched ---> You rub your hands together twenty times and focus on the feeling and the sound ---> You take five deep breaths ---> You remind yourself that his wife is sick and he's probably feeling stressed ---> You ignore his nasty comment and offer him a glass of iced tea

Can you see the difference?

In both cases, your brother acted like a jerk. The experience was the same. But in the first example, when you responded from an agitated nervous system, the whole thing went to you-know-where. In the second example, you were able to notice your rising emotional temperature and take action before your own tongue made things worse. You were able to take control of your response.

Experience X Response = Contentment

There are endless options for calming your nervous system once you identify that your temperature is rising. Everyone finds calm in a different place, but here are some common and useful approaches:

- Take ten slow, deep breaths. Focus all your attention on the feeling of breathing in and the feeling of breathing out.
- Pay attention to the sound of your breathing as you breathe in and as you breathe out.
- Count your breaths. With each breath in think "one," and with each breath out, think "calm." Repeat until you get to ten breaths.
- Rub the index finger and thumb of one hand together and focus on feeling the ridges of your fingers.
- Use your senses. Intentionally focus all your attention on what you see, what you hear, what you feel, what you smell, and what you taste.
- Pick up a small object and close your eyes. Focus all your attention on the feeling of that object. Note its heft, its shape, and its temperature. Notice if it is smooth, rough, or pointy. When your mind wanders, gently bring your attention back to your object.
- Take a hot bath and focus all your attention on the feel of the water, the smell of the soap, the slippery sensation between your fingers, and the sound the water makes when you move around.
- Pet your dog or cat and focus all your attention on the feeling of their fur.
- Turn on loud music and dance around your home.
- Run up and down the stairs or do jumping jacks to discharge some of your agitated energy.
- Put something tasty in your mouth but don't swallow it right

away. Focus all your attention on the feel of the food, the texture, the temperature, and the taste.

- Rub one hand over something with a strong texture like a wooden desk, a nubby couch, or a fluffy carpet. Focus all your attention on the sensations in your hand.
- Shake your arms to discharge your stress.
- Massage your temples and scalp.

Try several of these techniques and add some of your own.

In the beginning, these techniques may feel awkward or challenging or dumb. That's okay. Do them anyway. They work even if you don't believe in them. Just like lifting weights makes you stronger even if you don't think it will, practicing the calming of your stress response works even if you think the whole thing is silly. However, just like you won't be lifting seventy-five pounds on your first day in the gym, you won't be a self-calming master right out of the gate. The more you practice, the better it will work.

When you practice noticing your body's early stress warning alert and actively calm your agitated nervous system, you will get better and better at generating a neutral or positive response to a frustrating experience. This allows you to remain calmer and more balanced even when life is rough. This isn't a "life is a bunch of roses" or "God doesn't give you more than you can handle" sort of thing. It is not about being relentlessly positive. Rather, this approach changes your relationship with stressful events and gives you the tools to navigate them in a more effective way.

Could this approach have helped Carolina?

Carolina was frustrated with her dad's unhappiness and constant criticism, and furious that he wouldn't take her advice to engage more at his new facility so he could be happier and stop making her crazy. She was annoyed at her son who she thought was lazy and ungrateful. Carolina generally felt that everyone in her life expected her to help them, but no one cared enough to help her. She felt that life was unfair, and she always felt agitated and stressed.

When Carolina interacted with her dad and her son, they could feel her agitation. She was critical and angry at them, which made them upset and uninterested in making her feel better by taking her advice. Carolina's approach made her dad and her son dig in their heels more than they might have if she had approached them in a more neutral way.

Let's imagine a different scenario.

What if every time Andrew berated Carolina for not taking him out of the facility, she intentionally chose a self-reflective and self-calming approach. What if she noticed her chest and shoulders feeling tight and realized that she was getting agitated. What if instead of yelling at her dad, "If you'd just go to the activities, you'd be happier and stop complaining so much," she excused herself to the bathroom. What if she put cold water on her face, took four deep breaths, and rubbed her hands slowly together, feeling all the ridges on her palms, first with the right hand and then with the left. What if she shook her arms to discharge some of her stress and rubbed her temples with her thumbs.

Perhaps as she started to feel calmer, she might find empathy for her dad's frustration at growing old and being stuck in a place he didn't like. She might acknowledge her own feelings of guilt and consider writing about it in her journal or talking to a friend or therapist about it. Perhaps she would be able to tap into gratitude that she has a dad to fuss at or appreciate that he was being cared for in a good facility and she didn't need to worry about his safety. Or maybe she would notice how stressed she was and schedule weekly massages, or text some friends to ask if they wanted to go away on a weekend girls' trip.

Perhaps when Carolina went back out to her dad, she might have said something like, "Yeah dad, I'm sorry it sucks here. This must be really tough for you. Would you like to go out for ice cream?"

Experience X Response = Contentment

In Carolina's two examples, the experience of a cranky dad was the same. There isn't anything that Carolina can do to force her dad to be less cranky or to love his life. The only part of the equation that Carolina can control is her response. A more positive response creates more contentment for her, even if the original cranky pants doesn't improve at all.

Carolina can't change her dad, but she can change her response to him.

Getting command over your response to frustrating situations is a key skill to develop if you want to reduce your stress and improve your wellbeing. If you'd like help getting control of your response to stressful situations, contact us at www.CopingSupport.com. Send a message that says, "I'd like to get control of my response to stress" (or tell us what you'd like to accomplish) and you'll hear back from us with information about how we can help.

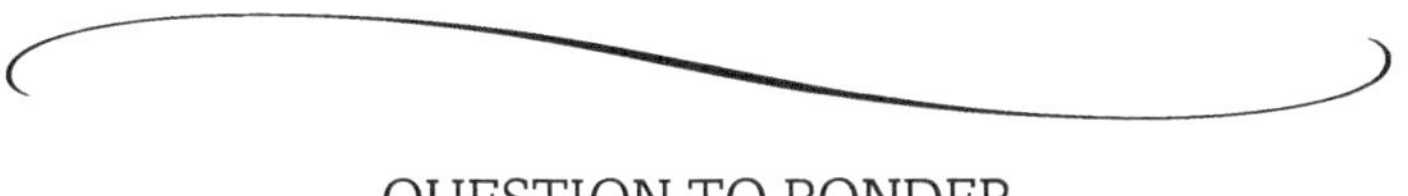

QUESTION TO PONDER

What situations in your life tend to agitate you?

FAMILY DISCUSSION QUESTION

Where do each of us feel stress in our body?

EXERCISE

Make a list of at least ten things that you can do to calm your nervous system when you get agitated.

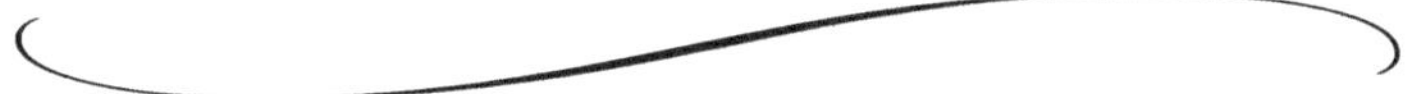

CHAPTER 11

Fill Your Cup

Helene was exhausted.

Her husband, Jon, had been battling amyotrophic lateral sclerosis (ALS) for six years, and Helene had been his devoted caregiver. ALS is a progressive neurodegenerative disease, and she had watched this beast steal bits of Jon's life little by little, until the man she had married was unrecognizable. Old Jon was a robust, bear-like man who loved to fix broken things and spend time outside. New Jon was bed bound and unable to bring a spoonful of pudding to his mouth.

Jon's speech was garbled, and he could no longer swallow safely. His mind was preserved, though, and so was his sarcastic sense of humor.

"He said he's sorry he didn't get the door for you," Helene told me.

I couldn't understand Jon's speech, but Helene still could.

"How rude of you," I said to Jon with a smile. He tried to smile back.

Jon and Helene were making the best of a terrible situation. They knew that his continued decline was inevitable, and they were both grieving for the life they used to live. They understood that ALS would eventually paralyze Jon's diaphragm, making him unable to breathe.

Helene and Jon had had some tough conversations. He had chosen her as his medical power of attorney and made it clear that when he was no longer able to breathe, he did not want to be hooked up to a breathing machine. He had gotten a feeding tube about a year before, when he'd started coughing after every meal, but that was as aggressive as he wanted to be. No more tubes. No ICU. No CPR. He just wanted medicines to keep himself comfortable.

Jon had decided to start hospice, which was how I ended up in his living room.

Helene spoke openly, in front of Jon, about how hard it had been on both of them.

"He was my rock," she said sadly.

Then she looked straight at Jon and said, "I loved our camping trips. Those were my favorite times."

He made an unintelligible noise that I took to mean, "Me too."

Helene looked at me then. "He's amazing. He's freaking amazing. If this were me going through this hell, I'd be having the world's biggest pity party. But Jon is just dealing with what comes." She turned to him, "I love you baby."

She wiped his tears and then her own with Jon's blanket. I wiped mine on my sleeve.

It wasn't just Jon's life that had become unrecognizable since the ALS diagnosis, Helene's life had become unrecognizable, too. Jon needed her to move him in bed so he wouldn't get bed sores, to hang the bag of liquid food that flowed into his stomach through a tube, and to wipe him after he pooped. They tried to approach this awful situation with affection, openness, and humor, but it wasn't easy.

They both got angry, occasionally at each other, and then they felt guilty. Sometimes each of them wished it was all over, but they didn't share that thought with each other.

Overall, though, they were both coping reasonably well with an unreasonably awful situation. They accepted what was coming. They realized that they wouldn't grow old together. They had talked about death, when Jon was still able, and he told Helene that he wasn't afraid.

As I talked with Helene, however, it struck me that her light seemed dim. She communicated openly, asked good questions, and wasn't agitated, but her energy was flat. Her flame was flickering and seemed at risk of being snuffed out. I assessed her for depression, but that wasn't the problem.

Helene wasn't depressed, she was depleted. Her emotional, physical, and spiritual "cup" was simply empty.

"Helene," I said. "This has been rough on you, hasn't it?"

"You have no idea," she said slowly. Her head moved almost imperceptibly back and forth, and she sighed through puffed cheeks. "No one understands the hell that we live every day."

"Tell me about the hardest parts," I said.

She was quiet for a long time. I got the sense that so much of it was hard, that my question seemed unanswerable.

She landed on, "I've lost myself."

"Tell me more about that," I answered gently.

She led me into the other room.

Helene shared that she had transformed from a quirky, funny, artistic, social person into a nurse who worked twenty-four/seven with no pay and no vacation days. She had been trying to keep a positive attitude for Jon, but it was getting noticeably harder.

"It's just so much of the same," she said. "Doctors and medicines and tube feeds and bed baths. Over and over. Every day is the same."

"What do you do when you get a break?" I asked her, knowing exactly what she was going to say.

"What's a break?" she joked with a smirk.

She shook her head slowly and looked at the floor. She seemed far away. I stayed quiet and let the silence bloom. I imagined her remembering the woman that she used to be and the life that she used to live.

Eventually she looked up with a little laugh-snort and shook her head a few times. "Anyway . . . ," she said, "It is what it is."

Unsurprisingly, Helene wasn't sleeping well, wasn't exercising, and wasn't having any fun.

"I'm too exhausted to do anything except care for Jon," she said, "And how could I possibly go have fun when he's home suffering? There's no way I could do that."

Helene was loving, committed, attentive, and accepting. She was also hanging on by her fingernails, and about to crash to the ground in a heap. Helene was depleted. She was empty. Her cup was bone dry.

Being depleted is not the same as being sad.

You can be terribly sad but not depleted, and you can be depleted for many reasons other than sadness. We couldn't fix Helene's sadness, but we could, and should, work on filling up her empty cup.

Why?

Because life's challenges, from tiny ones to monstrous ones, are *more* challenging when your cup is empty. Life is simply harder with an empty cup.

Since you're reading this book, I'm going to assume that your cup is emptier than it could be. Caregiving, or even caring about someone who is ill, is the equivalent of poking a hole in the bottom of your paper cup and watching the iced tea, beer, or Chardonnay pour out onto the floor. If you don't take some action, there will be nothing left in that cup to keep you going.

I like the metaphor of a cup because it reminds me of a cozy coffee mug or a decorative teacup, and those things make me happy. If you'd rather imagine a gas tank or a tea pot or a bathtub, feel free to insert your favorite metaphor. But no matter what you call it, you need to gauge the fluid level in your vessel and take steps to keep it more than half full.

The Causes of an Empty Cup

If you fill a cup with water, leave it on the counter, and come back in a few weeks, what will you find? You'll probably find an empty cup. But how did it get empty? Assuming that no one snuck in and poured out all the water, there are two possibilities. Or maybe three. Either the water eventually evaporated and no one filled it back up from the top, or there was a leak in the cup and the water drained out from the bottom. The third possibility is that both things happened at once.

So, when we ponder the idea of how to fill up your cup, we have to consider what could fill it from the top and what could be emptying it from the bottom. Both parts of the cup equation are important.

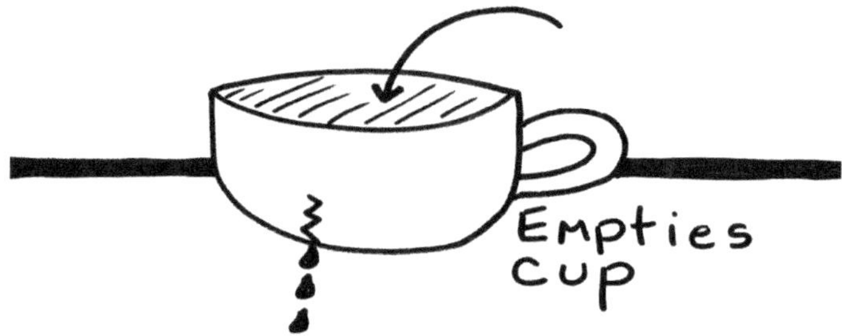

There's a key concept that I don't want you to miss: one person's cup emptier is another person's cup filler. So it isn't about the action, it's about how the action works for you. For example, some people love running. It energizes them, makes them feel strong, and it powerfully fills their cup. Other people find running as pleasurable as having a toenail removed and if you made them run, everything in their cup would immediately drain out. Some people love yoga, and it fills their cup. For other people, yoga makes them feel uncomfortable and awkward and generally miserable. You may have had people tell you that you should meditate. For people who like meditation, it's a wonderful healing tool. For others it can feel frustrating and dumb. What fills my cup might empty yours.

For this reason, no one can decide how another person should fill their cup. It is a highly personal experience. So, the goal is for you to figure out what fills and empties *your* cup.

What Empties Your Cup?

Let's consider the cup emptiers first.

Since everyone is different, I don't know what empties your cup. Maybe you don't know either, although you probably have an inkling about it. But I can give you a list of things that tend to be cup emptiers. See if any of these should be on your list:

- Overscheduling
- Not sleeping enough
- Not moving enough
- Difficult people
- Negative self-talk
- A messy house or office
- Work you don't like
- Guilt
- Anxiety

- Untreated depression
- Pain or other symptoms
- Not asking for help
- Illness
- Arguing
- Procrastinating
- Financial concerns
- Chronic worrying
- Too much TV or screen time
- Overeating
- Overuse of alcohol, cannabis, or illegal drugs
- Eating a non-nutritious diet
- Smoking
- Shame
- Regret
- Being oversensitive to criticism
- Being dehydrated
- Having unrealistic expectations of yourself
- Having unrealistic expectations of other people
- Grief or anticipatory grief
- Having a pessimistic worldview
- Having poor boundaries
- A history of psychological abuse or trauma

You may have noticed that some of the cup emptiers are out of your control. You can't simply decide not to have an illness or childhood trauma or grief. You can't even necessarily control the difficult people in your life because they may share a gene pool, or even a roll of toilet paper, with you. While it is helpful to look at all of your cup emptiers, even if they aren't changeable, pay special attention to the behaviors, attitudes, people, or activities that empty your cup and are within your control. Draw yourself a cup and write all your cup emptiers on the bottom.

Here's an example:

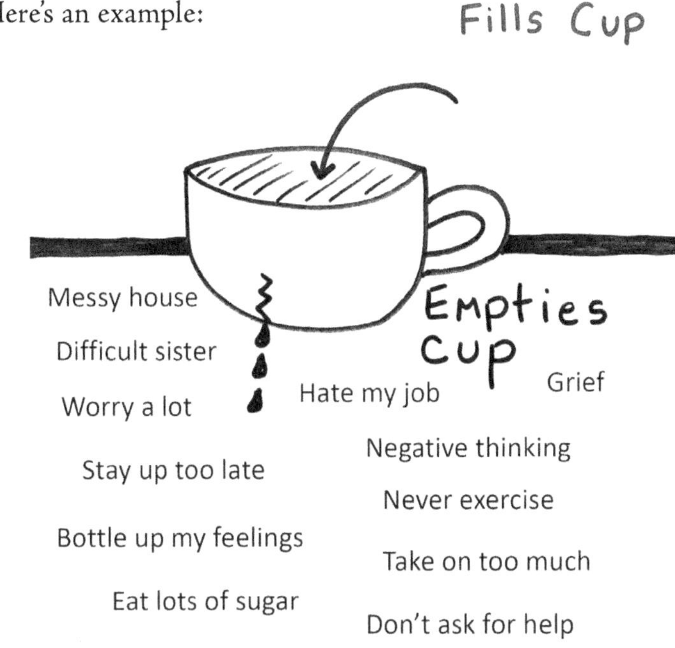

Then pick two or three of the changeable cup emptiers that you are willing to work on. This person might pick "take on too much" and "stay up too late," or "eat lots of sugar" and "don't ask for help." Circle the ones that you are willing to work on that will give you the most benefit.

A note for the over-achievers and perfectionists: you probably want to make a list of fifteen cup emptiers and work on all of them starting today. No. That is against the rules. You can only pick three things to work on, and two would be even better. You can come back for more in a month or two once you've mastered the two that you're starting to work on today.

What Fills Your Cup?

Just like everyone has their own cup emptiers, cup fillers are personal, too. For some people cooking is a cup filler, while for other people it's a big snore chore. Some people love walking the dog and others resent every steamy bag of poop. This is not about what you think you *should* do, or should like, it is about what floats your particular boat.

This list may give you some ideas, but your cup fillers are all your own.

- Seven hours of sleep every night
- Regular vacations
- Going for walks
- Playing with your pets
- Hanging out with your kids
- Reading a book
- Watching funny movies
- Spending time with friends
- Baking
- Creating things
- Going to the gym
- Hugs
- Yoga
- Tai Chi
- Getting a massage
- Journaling
- Being alone
- Making or listening to music
- Writing
- Qi gong
- Running
- Learning things
- An uncluttered environment
- A daily gratitude ritual
- Gardening
- Archery
- Traveling
- Volunteering
- Being kind to yourself

- Teaching
- Organizing things
- A steaming cup of coffee or tea
- Setting boundaries
- Seeing a therapist
- Resting

Now add your particular cup fillers to your cup picture. It might look something like this:

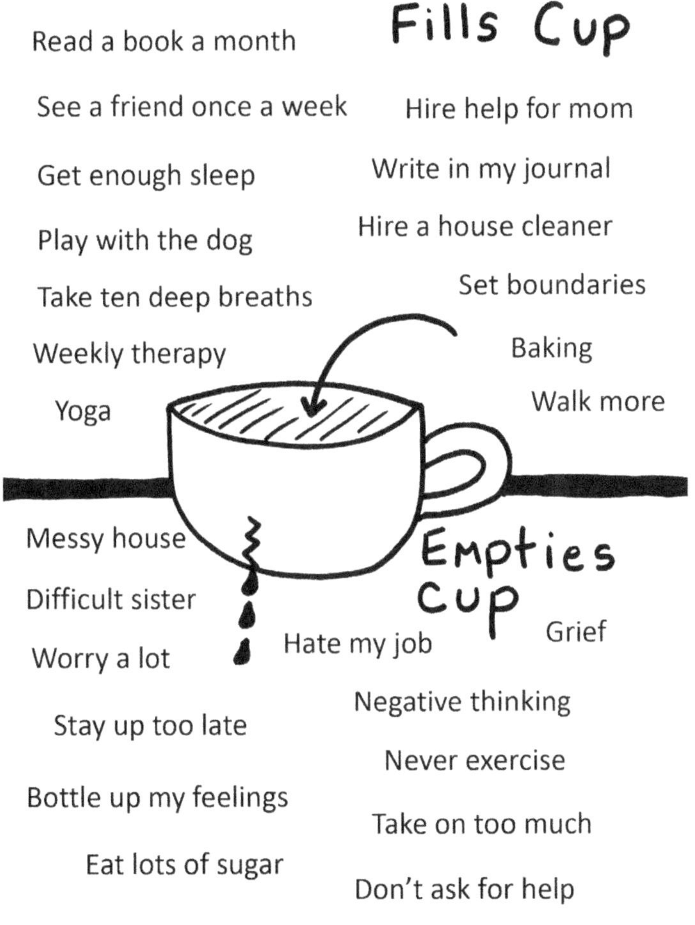

Choose two or three cup fillers that you can add to your life. Can you hire a house cleaner, get an aide to help care for your loved one, and get to bed on time? Can you sign up for yoga, walk every evening after dinner, and see a friend once a week?

I see you, over-achievers. Just two or three things. No more.

So draw yourself that cup, fill out the emptiers and the fillers, and circle two to three of each that you are going to start to work on. This gives you four to six clear changes that you can make, starting immediately, to start to fill your cup back up.

Sometimes, when things are feeling particularly bleak, it can be hard to come up with any cup fillers at all. If that sounds like you, don't worry. This is common and understandable. The trick in this situation is to remember a time when your life seemed to be going better. What were the things that you did way back then? Did you exercise or meditate or bake cookies for the neighbors? Did you read or paint or go to concerts? Which of those things lifted your spirits? What did you enjoy? What made you happy? Connecting to the past version of you that was happier than today's version can give you some ideas for how to fill your cup.

One cup filler that deserves a special call-out is intentional gratitude. Gratitude gets a bad rap for being cliché or masquerading as toxic positivity, but a well-done gratitude ritual is a supercharged cup filler that is worth exploring.

The idea of a gratitude ritual is simply to intentionally focus on the good things that are happening in your life, even if you feel like you're in the middle of a tornado. A gratitude ritual does not in any way negate all the crappy things that you are facing. Not at all. It is simply a decision to pivot your attention to something that is kind of okay. There are different techniques for using gratitude to fill your cup (see below), but I recommend that you at least incorporate a brief daily gratitude ritual into your routine. See page 175 for ideas of things that you might be grateful for.

Using Gratitude to Support Wellbeing

Daily Gratitude Ritual

1. Choose your number
   - How long will your daily list be? Will you call to mind three things that you're grateful for? Five things? Even noticing one thing per day for which you are grateful is a great start.
   - Make them different every day
   - If you choose the same three things to be grateful for every day, they will eventually lose their punch. Also, you won't be training yourself to find new good things even in hard times. Your daily "gratefuls" can be large or small, they just can't be the same as the ones from the day before.

2. Choose your plan
   - Will you write your gratitude list in a journal? Think it to yourself as you lay in bed or brush your teeth or take a shower? Share it out loud with another person? Text it to a friend? Record it on your phone? There is no one right way. The best way is the one that you'll do.

3. Check in with yourself
   - Did you start a gratitude journal but end up not liking it? Did your gratitude buddy flake out? Do you fall asleep before you can complete your list? Give yourself permission to modify your plan until you find one that works. And if you do one for a while and get bored with it, change it up. Generating the list is what is important, the mechanics don't matter at all.

4. Give yourself grace
   - You will forget to do your gratitude list. I'm sure of it. And that is totally okay. The goal is to do it daily-ish, but if this is a new habit it will take time to establish and that's just fine. Reminders can be helpful, such as sticky notes around the house or an alert on your smartphone; just be sure not to give up simply because you aren't perfect. If you forget for a few days and then remember, one of your 'gratefuls' for that day can be that you remembered to do your gratitude ritual.

Gratitude List

- A gratitude list is a once-in-a-while way to use gratitude.
- Grab your journal or a piece of notebook paper or the inside cover of this book.
- Write down every single thing that you can think of that you are grateful for. It should be a long list.
- When you run out of things to write, don't stop. What about the third-grade teacher who saw greatness in you when you felt invisible? Or that cool trip that you took. Or your sense of humor. Or your symmetrical eyebrows. Write it all down. Everything. People, experiences, conveniences, accomplishments, personal qualities, childhood pets, and favorite desserts.
- Once you can't possibly think of one more thing, read the list to yourself and ruminate on all the good things that have happened in your life.

Gratitude Letter

- A gratitude letter is a heartfelt letter written to a person, living, dead, or fictional, explaining how they have helped you in your life. Pour your heart out in this letter. It is the feelings that matter, not the prose.
- If you can, read the letter out loud to your person. I know that this might sound scary or uncomfortable, but it can be a powerful experience. If your person is no longer living, or you can't access them directly, read the letter out loud in front of another person who you trust. If another person isn't available, read the letter out loud to yourself.

Things You Might Be Grateful For

- People—current and past, living and deceased, loved ones but also neighbors from childhood, teachers, or your favorite barista
- Experiences—study abroad, research projects, summer camp, fishing with your dad, vacations
- Comforts—heat, a functioning car, a comfy bed, air conditioning, toilets that work
- Pets—current and past
- Natural world—flowers, space, sea animals
- Religious or spiritual connections—relationship with a deity, spiritual community, prayer ritual
- Foods—coffee, pasta, a smoothie in the morning
- Possessions—beloved jewelry, your favorite blanket, a flat screen TV
- Hobbies—gardening, sewing, fly fishing, hiking, photography, wood working
- Talents—acting, singing, visual arts, yodeling, skateboarding
- Athletics—participating or observing
- Exercise—running, aerobics, boxing
- Personality traits—deep empathy, sense of humor, adventurous spirit
- Self-care rituals—yoga, tai chi, meditation, facials
- Your body—legs that can run, the ability to sleep, cancer in remission, pain under control, great hair

I tried to keep a gratitude journal, but I just couldn't keep it up. I would mean to do it every night before bed but then I'd be tired or forget, and I'd beat myself up about it the next day. "You can't even take five minutes to write down what you're grateful for?"

It isn't the form of the daily gratitude practice that matters, luckily for me, it is the regularity. Some days you could write in a journal, if you like that sort of thing, and other days you could mention your 'gratefuls' to your spouse at breakfast or share with a friend by phone or just call them to mind when you're in the shower.

For a while I had a gratitude ritual with a childhood friend. Every day we texted each other five things that we were grateful for from that day or the day before. No commentary, just five things. This was important because we might not have had time to engage in a whole conversation, but we certainly had the time to text five words or phrases. I might text:

1. Coffee
2. My chihuahua
3. A nice conversation with one of my daughters
4. Air conditioning
5. The tomatoes in my garden

And she might reply with:
1. Sitting at Starbucks
2. A cooler day than normal
3. Fun at the dog park
4. Finished an art project
5. A good conversation with a friend from work

I loved this practice. It was good for accountability, and we got a window into each other's worlds from across the country. I'm not sure why we stopped. We should probably start it up again.

I have had many iterations of my gratitude practice over the years. Lately my practice is just in my own head. Every night I call to mind five things that I'm grateful for from the day as I lay in bed to go to sleep. I like this practice because it offers a positive sheen on the day, no matter how it has gone.

Gratitude is entirely distinct from toxic positivity, which tries to whitewash an entire day or month or experience. Gratitude, on the other hand, is simply stepping over the poop in search of the flowers. Even on a heartbreaking day, a cuddle from my dog can give me a moment of comfort. Even if I've been crying, coffee still tastes good.

Your Cup Meter

I suggest that you keep an eye on the fullness of your cup. Be sure to check the meter on a regular basis. Once a day might be too often, but once a week could work. Your cup is getting low? Pick a few emptiers to do less of and a few fillers to do more of.

When your cup is empty it feels awful. It feels exhausting and depleting and sometimes even hopeless or stuck. Keeping an eye on the meter and noticing when your levels are low gives you an opportunity to take action to fix the problem before it becomes a crisis.

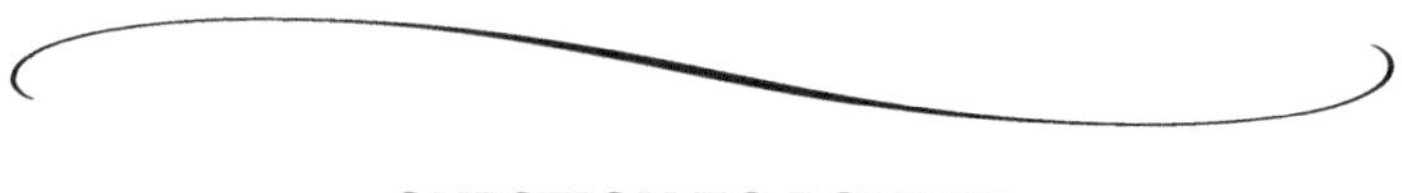

QUESTION TO PONDER

If you were to start a gratitude ritual, what would it look like?

FAMILY DISCUSSION QUESTION

What do we do that empties each other's cups? What change could we make to help each other's cups stay full?

EXERCISE

Draw a cup and add your cup emptiers and cup fillers. Circle two or three of each that you plan to work on starting this week.

PAUSE BREAK

Take two slow, deep breaths.

Call to mind a specific time in your life when
you felt the experience of love or awe.

This could be a time when you were little or the love you
feel for a child or pet. It could be the way you feel when you
see a waterfall, a vast ocean, or a beautiful night sky.

When you've chosen your image, close your eyes and
spend a few moments fully experiencing the feeling
of love or awe. Notice where you feel it in your body.

When you're ready, open your eyes.

Take two slow, deep breaths.

PART 3

Nurture Authentic and Meaningful Connections

CHAPTER 12

Master Courageous Conversations

Ellie caught me in the hallway on my way in to see her mom, Mona, who had been admitted to the hospital for worsening congestive heart failure. Mona was seventy-nine but she seemed older. She had had six hospitalizations in less than a year, and with each one she became more frail and less independent. Ellie knew that Mona's doctor had consulted palliative care, and she wanted to catch me before I could get to her mom.

"Don't say anything negative," Ellie told me forcefully. "We don't want to upset her, and we don't want to take away her hope."

Ellie's body language was tense. Her whole upper body looked like she was preparing for a fight, but I could sense that what looked like anger was probably fear. Ellie loved her mom, and she was trying to protect her.

"Tell me more about your mom," I said.

"She is our whole world, and we know she can get through this," Ellie replied. She sounded like a school principal scolding a student. "I don't want you scaring her or telling her that things are bad."

The problem was things *were* bad. Mona's heart had been progressively failing for some time and her decline had, unfortunately, sped up over the last few months. Her heart was getting weaker, her kidneys weren't functioning well, and she was quickly losing the ability to live independently.

Her doctors had done all the right things. They had adjusted Mona's medication, counseled her to eat less salt, and offered suggestions for how to keep her safer at home. She had had ultrasounds of her heart, seen multiple cardiologists, and taken plenty of medications.

I asked Ellie what she thought about her mom's condition. "She is strong, and she can handle anything," Ellie said. "We know she'll get better."

When I started to express my concern about her progression Ellie stopped me. "I don't want to hear any negativity," she said.

I spent some time with Mona, Ellie, and Mona's other daughter, Alana. Ellie did most of the talking. I determined that Mona was fully oriented and able to understand her medical condition, and I made a mental note to return later to chat with Mona alone.

When I came back, Mona's daughters had gone home. I sat at her bedside, and she seemed eager to talk. She told me about her life, what had been most important to her, and how much she adored her daughters. The three of them had always been close, she told me, and she knew that her illness was hard on them.

"Ellie's the bossy one," she told me with a laugh. "I know she's just trying to protect me, but she's making us all a little crazy. I know that things don't look good, but she doesn't seem to want to accept that."

"Have you told Ellie what you're thinking, about how things are going?" I asked Mona.

"No, not really," Mona said. "I don't want to rile her up, so I've just kept my mouth shut."

"How do you feel about that?" I asked.

"I don't know," Mona said with a sigh. "I feel kind of all alone with it, you know? I know what's coming but I can't talk about it with my kids."

"That sounds lonely," I said. "And maybe scary?"

"I don't feel scared," Mona told me, "But lonely. Yeah. It's lonely. And it's sad. I want to be able to share what's going on with my people, you know? I don't want to go through this all by myself."

Ellie didn't mean to make her mom feel lonely and sad. She thought she was protecting her mom and shielding her from sadness. Ellie didn't realize that Mona was thinking about her own physical decline and coming to a sense of acceptance about her mortality. Ellie was able to shut the reality of her mom's illness out of her mind, but Mona couldn't do that. So entirely without meaning to, Ellie left her beloved mother to face her mortality all by herself.

Now, let's not be too hard on Ellie. She was experiencing anticipatory grief and was terribly sad about what was happening to her mom. It's hard to face hard things. But here's the problem: by running from the unfortunate reality that Mona's life was coming to an end, Ellie was reducing the amount of closeness that she could experience with her mom while she was still alive. Just as in-person connection with her mom was becoming most vital, Ellie was putting unnecessary space between them.

If Ellie understood this, she might make an intentional attempt to bridge this gap. She might ask Mona questions such as:

- "How do you feel things are going with your health overall?"
- "Do you ever think about what would happen if you get worse?"
- "Is there anything that you'd like to talk about?"
- "Is there anything that you'd like to ask me?"
- "Do you ever think about dying?"
- "Are you scared?"

She could also simply say something like:
- "I just want you to know that you can talk to me about anything. Even hard things. Even things that you think people don't talk about."

This would make it clear to Mona that she didn't need to face this time all by herself. She might not choose to talk about it with Ellie, but just knowing that she could, if she wanted to, would be comforting.

Talking About Advancing Illness or Mortality

It can be extremely hard, scary, uncomfortable, and sad to talk with your ill loved one about the progression of their illness or the possibility that it will take their life. It's just hard. No one wants to do it.

There might even be a tiny voice in your head telling you that if you don't talk about it, it isn't real. I wish it worked like that. If avoiding talking about bad things kept them from happening, no one would lose their job, get left by their spouse, or lose their life.

The reality is that not talking about your loved one's impending mortality doesn't keep them on Earth longer, but it may negatively impact the time that they have left.

If your loved one's illness is severe, life-threatening, and progressive, you and other people in your life are undoubtedly suffering. I wish you didn't have to walk this road. I wish that I had a magic wand to give you that could make it all go away.

But since I don't, let's talk about how to talk about it.

The 'D' Word

Saying "death" or "dying" does not make people die.

Are you with me on this? You may not even realize it if you harbor this idea deep in your psyche, but many people do. Many people feel a sense of dark magic surrounding the word death, like it needs to be said in a whisper or behind a hand covering your mouth. Like if we say "death" or "dying" somebody is going to die.

That's not how dying works.

Death is heavy and sad and profoundly bizarre. The idea that a person can be here and then not be here is completely mind-blowing and unfathomable. It is not something to make light of.

Yet it is part of the deal. We are born onto this planet, we find experiences and connections and love, and then we have to go. That's just the way this game is played. I don't know why it works this way, but it does. And it works this way for every single one of us. Everyone you know. Everyone I know. Everyone.

So, while death is sad and distressing and nothing that we want to talk about, it is part of life. And because it is part of life, we need to be able to talk about it. We don't have to like it, but we should learn the skills and gather the courage to do it when we need to. If someone that you love wants to talk to you about their advancing illness, their goals of care, or their feelings about dying, I suggest that you take a deep breath, pull up a chair, and open your heart to the conversation. You may not want to do this, and that's okay. Do it anyway. This is important, and it isn't about what feels comfortable, it's about what would ease your loved one's journey.

This is soul work.

You don't need to have any special skills to have these conversations. You just need to show up and breathe. And then you need to share your empathy, your kindness, your vulnerability, and your willingness to explore the inexplicable mystery of human life.

The energy that you bring to these conversations matters much more than the words.

That said, it can be helpful to have some words in mind. Here are some examples:

For people with advancing illness

- "Do you ever think about what the future might bring?"
- "Does anything make you worried or scared?"
- "Is there anything that you'd like me to know?"
- "Is there something that you'd like to talk about?"
- "Do you ever think about dying? Are you afraid?"

If the doctor suggests hospice

- "Your doctor said that we should think about starting hospice. We don't have to decide today, but let's talk about it so we know all our options."
- "Hospice is all about making you feel better and reducing your pain and other symptoms that are making it hard for you to enjoy your life. They are the experts in managing pain, nausea, and all the other stuff that comes along with your condition. They have doctors, nurses, social workers, chaplains, home health aides, and volunteers to support us all through this tough time. Also, they have on call people, so if we have any trouble in the middle of the night, we can call them and they'll come to the house to help us if we need it. It's covered by insurance. Should we talk to them to learn more?"

For people who don't have an advance directive

- "I would love for us to talk about filling out our advance directives. Let's all do it together. I'll print out the forms, and we can talk about each of the questions and then each fill out our own form. How does that sound?"
- Note: Chapter four covers advance directives in depth. You can find an advance directive online by searching "advance directive" and the name of your state.

For people who are filling out an advance directive

- "We have to think about what we would want if we were ever in a coma and not expected to wake up or if we were coming to the end of our lives. Would we want CPR or to be hooked up to a breathing machine? Would we want to be kept alive with a feeding tube in our stomach if we weren't expected to wake up or recover? Basically, which is more important to us: living every day possible no matter what shape we're in, or focusing on being awake and able to communicate? It's a quantity vs. quality thing."

For people who need to decide on their "code status" (whether or not they want CPR or breathing machine support if their heart or lungs were to stop working)

- "To make a decision about your 'code status' you need to think about two things: your health situation and what your goals are. The question is, what do you want the doctors to do if your heart stops or you're unable to breathe? Because of (your serious medical condition), there's a chance that if your heart or lungs stopped working, the doctors couldn't bring you all the way back. So, there's a risk that you'd get stuck on a breathing machine and couldn't get off. Should we ask the doctors how likely it is that CPR or a breathing tube would help you come back to how you are now? Or have you already decided what you want to do?"
- "You know, even if you choose "Do Not Resuscitate (DNR)" you can still get all kinds of medical treatments like heart medicine, antibiotics, blood transfusions, etc. It doesn't mean that they stop treating you."

For people who have chosen aggressive potentially life-prolonging treatments and don't want hospice or palliative care

- "It isn't time for hospice now since you want to continue with (*medical treatments such as chemotherapy or weekly blood transfusions*), but you can still benefit from palliative care. Hospice is for when you've stopped aggressive medically focused treatments and want to focus on aggressive symptom-focused treatments. But palliative care is for anyone with a serious illness who has symptoms, stress, or decisions to make. Palliative care helps reduce your symptoms (like pain and nausea), helps the whole family cope, and helps you make important medical decisions. You can get palliative care even if you're getting medically focused care and hoping to prolong your life."

For people who are ill and are trying to figure out exactly how much aggressive medical care they still want

- Note: I explain the POLST/MOLST below so don't get freaked out by all the letters. The POLST and MOLST are the same form; different states call them different things.
- "There is something called a POLST (Physician Order for Life-Sustaining Treatment) or MOLST (Medical Order for Life Sustaining Treatment) that can help you communicate your wishes to your doctors in case you ever aren't able to tell them yourself. I got the form from the doctor. Can we look over the form together and discuss what you'd want us to do if you were to get sicker?"
- "Even if you have an advance directive, if your illness is getting serious you should also have a POLST/MOLST."

It is important to understand the difference between an advance directive and a POLST/MOLST. An advance directive is a guide for the theoretical future that is signed by the person themself. It is designed to tell your loved ones and your medical providers how you generally feel about prolonging your life if you were to be in a persistent vegetative state, very ill, or close to death. People usually fill these out long before there is a medical emergency. They are so important that all of chapter four is dedicated to advance directives. An advance directive is not a medical order, but physicians and other healthcare providers are ethically obligated to use it as a guide when they are deciding how to treat you. The exception is that EMTs are obligated to treat you as aggressively as possible unless you have a

POLST/MOLST signed by the doctor that tells them not to. They can't use an advance directive for this purpose. Everyone should have an advance directive and you should review it every year or so. As I mentioned before, my husband and I have advance directives, and both of my young adult daughters have them, too. You may think that young people don't need them, but I strongly disagree. Young people can be tragically injured in accidents, and they deserve to determine in advance if they would want their life artificially prolonged if they were never expected to recover.

A POLST/MOLST, on the other hand, is more appropriate for people who are currently facing an advanced serious illness. It is a medical order that is signed by the physician, physician assistant, or nurse practitioner after an in-depth conversation with the patient, and it is much more specific than an advance directive. In addition to communicating if a patient will get CPR or mechanical breathing support if their heart or lungs stop working, or a feeding tube if they are unable to feed themselves, the POLST/MOLST clarifies if the patient wants dialysis, hospitalization, antibiotics, medical testing, or blood transfusions.

This is not an all-or-nothing situation. In between "do everything" and "do nothing" there is an important sea of nuance. Your loved one might want to return to the hospital for antibiotics if they get a urinary tract infection even though they do not want CPR or mechanical breathing support. They might want dialysis if their fragile kidneys fail, but not want to be kept alive with a feeding tube if they have a stroke and are unable to care for themselves or recognize their family. There is also an option to choose a short trial of a certain intervention, such as mechanical breathing support, but discontinue it if the physicians do not expect the person to recover.

The POLST/MOLST form is very clear and can be an excellent tool to help you start a conversation with your loved one about their wishes for treatment if their condition were to decline. You can get the form from your primary care doctor, geriatrician, or hospital doctor, and you can find the form yourself by searching MOLST or POLST and your state. If you get the form yourself, be sure to bring it to your doctor to sign it. Then you can keep copies in the house, in your purse, with your loved one's papers, and at the hospital where your loved one is most likely to go if they need emergency care. Your loved one's medical power of attorney should have a copy, too.

Things You Should Know About Hospice and Palliative Care

- Both hospice and palliative care are provided by physicians and other clinicians who have special training and expertise in managing pain and other symptoms.
- Palliative care is whole person care for families facing serious illness, focused on relieving pain and suffering.
- You can have palliative care alongside aggressive life-prolonging care.
- Palliative care physicians are Board certified in their specialty just like cardiologists, neurologists, and other specialists.
- All hospice is palliative care, but not all palliative care is hospice.
- Hospice is appropriate in the last six months of a person's life, while people can have palliative care for many years.
- You can have some standard medical interventions while on hospice. Examples include oral antibiotics, occasional blood transfusions, and even radiation if it is used to manage pain. Each hospice will make its own determination about what they can provide. Hospice does NOT mean stopping care.
- You can choose hospice and then stop it at any time if you choose to. It isn't a permanent decision.
- Some people "graduate" from hospice if their medical condition stabilizes.

Fears of Death

Sometimes, your loved one might share with you that they are afraid of dying. This may be distressing for you to hear, and it can be hard to know how to respond. "Oh, don't worry about that" is the wrong response, but what is the right response? The best immediate response is some version of "I'm here." You could express this in words, such as "I'll be with you no matter what," with a hug, a hand squeeze, an understanding head nod, or even with silence and a few slow deep breaths.

When you're ready to dive in a little more deeply, it can be helpful to know exactly what they are afraid of, because there might be something that you can do to allay their fears. Fears of death generally fall into three categories.

1. Fear of the Process

Sometimes people are afraid of what death will feel like. They worry that they'll have uncontrolled pain, shortness of breath, or anxiety. They might worry that they won't get good medical care or that no one will help them with their symptoms. Basically, they are afraid that they will suffer.

Response: If your loved one is afraid of the *process* of dying, this is a great opportunity to introduce the idea of palliative care and hospice. Palliative care and hospice clinicians are experts in symptom management for people with serious illnesses. Having a hospice team support your loved one near the end of their life can dramatically reduce the chance that they will have uncontrolled pain or other distressing symptoms.

2. Fear that you won't be okay

This one can be tough. You may also feel like you won't be okay. It's important to clarify exactly what your loved one means when they say this. They may mean that they worry that you will fall apart, or they may mean that you don't know the computer passwords, how to fix the glitchy garbage disposal, or what school supplies to buy.

Response: If they are worried about the more practical side of life, there is a simple intervention to ease their mind: create a manual. I have seen patients visibly and profoundly relax after sharing the important practical details that they've been storing in their head. You could interview them and write down the details, record their instructions on your phone, or give them a pad and a pen to jot down details as they think of them. Some people want an organized notebook with tabs, but others are just as satisfied with a legal pad and a pencil.

If your loved one is afraid that you will emotionally fall apart without them, your approach will be different. It is fine if your response to this one is simply a big hug, but if you feel up it, there are some things that you can do to lighten their burden. The first, and the hardest, is to reassure them that you and your family will be okay. You might say something like, "We will miss you so much and our hearts will be broken when you go, but we'll lean on each other, and we will eventually be okay."

Gathering family at your loved one's bedside to deliver this message as a group can be a powerful experience, but it works just as well one on one. Don't worry if you don't feel up to doing this. It's okay if you do it, and it's okay if you don't.

3. Fear of what happens after death

If your loved one is worried about what happens after death, it is time to call in reinforcements. This is a form of spiritual distress and there are people who specialize in this exact situation.

Response: Offering to arrange for your loved one to talk about their concerns with someone trained to address spiritual distress is generally the best approach. Non-denominational chaplains can be found in hospitals, palliative care organizations, and hospices, and they can be great comfort to people suffering with spiritual distress. If your loved one would like to speak to a religious leader from their own faith, that's another good option. If a spiritual leader is not a good fit, a therapist or grief counselor may also be helpful.

Tips For Making Tough Conversations Easier

1. Do it Messy

These conversations aren't easy. You probably don't want to have them, and you may not feel like you have what it takes to skillfully lead a challenging conversation. That's fine. Do it anyway. It is the heart and intention that matter more than the words. You can be awkward, flushed, and stuttering and still provide healing. Simply being willing to enter into the muck with someone you care about can be a meaningful and enriching experience for them, and a moment of deep understanding and connection for you.

2. Bring Your Healing Presence

Energy is contagious. If you bring angry or frustrated energy to a courageous conversation it is unlikely to go well, and if you bring tight and buttoned up energy your loved one is less likely to vulnerably share themself with you. This doesn't mean that you have to have it all together. In fact, the opposite is true. Bringing your messy, open, vulnerable realness may allow your loved one to do the same. It doesn't always work this way, but it is certainly worth the effort.

Before you enter into a tough conversation, check in with your own self first. Take some slow, deep breaths. Shake out the tension in your arms. Close your eyes and take a moment to center yourself. Say a prayer if that's your thing. Imagine your heart filling with love and compassion. See if you can make your very presence a healing experience for your loved one, even before you say a word.

3. Use Reflective Listening

Most of us spend a large portion of our lives trying to be heard. Yet your average person would get a C-minus in listening skills. Often when one person is talking, even if they are baring their soul, the listener is only half listening because they are already formulating their response. This is why reflective listening is so powerful.

When you use reflective listening, you simply reflect back to the person what you heard. Even in heavy conversations, this approach is usually enthusiastically received because it just feels so good to be truly heard and understood.

If your loved one says:
"You know, this is really getting to be too much. I'm tired of being in pain and I'm tired of trying to fight the inevitable. I've lived a great life and I'm not afraid of whatever is next."

You might say:
"It sounds like you feel like you don't want to fight or have pain anymore. You aren't afraid and you're ready for whatever is next."

Then add my favorite question:
"Did I get that right?"

Let's try another one.

If your loved one says:
"I'm sick of everyone treating me like I'm an invalid. I know everything that's going on and you all need to stop treating me like I don't."

You might say:

"It sounds like you're getting annoyed at us because we're treating you like you're sick and you just want to be treated like yourself. Did I get that right?"

If you want to step it up a notch, you can reflect back the emotions that you think the person is expressing even if they don't explicitly say the words. Here's what that might look like.

If your loved one says:

"Can you believe that the nurse did that? And the doctor too? What is wrong with this stupid place?"

You might say:

"It sounds like you're really angry about how things are going."

Don't be concerned that you'll misinterpret what the person is saying. You might, but it's okay. If you got it wrong the person will usually say something like, "No, I'm not angry, I'm just shocked that they would do that."

I've never had anyone be upset at me for getting it wrong. They simply correct you, but they still feel like you're trying hard to understand how they feel.

You might be thinking that this sounds dumb. Or that you will annoy the heck out of your person if you talk to them this way. I used to think that too, until I started regularly using reflective listening. The crazy thing is that even if you repeat back exactly what the person said to you, if you do it with the sincere attempt to understand what they are communicating, it is almost always well received.

Some common ways to start a reflective listening statement are:

- "What I hear you saying is . . ."
- "If I understood you correctly . . ."
- "It seems like . . ."
- "It sounds like . . ."

Don't worry if you feel awkward about using this technique at first. That's normal. The more you do it the easier it gets, and the more you practice the more easily you can integrate the words into your own natural way of speaking.

4. Use Silence Strategically

Silence can be terrifying. I'm not sure why, but we seem to have all learned that if there is a void, someone had better fill it with noise. Yet when you start to think about silence in a new way, you will begin to appreciate its beauty and its power. There is a sense of pause in silence. A chance to catch your breath. The opportunity to notice a bird chirping outside the window or the thrum of an air conditioner. There is space for slower breaths in silence, for unclenching your jaw and straightening your spine. In silence, there is space for thoughts to bloom and emotions to process.

I encourage you to play with silence. Allow it to be one of your communication tools. When you ask a question and your person takes time to answer, try your very hardest not to fill the space. If a heavy thought or comment or issue is in the air, leave some room for the related thoughts, feelings, or insights to unfold. Sitting in silence with someone that you care about can be a more intimate experience than filling the room with words.

5. Watch for Flares and Listen for Clues

Sometimes people who are thinking about their own mortality will send out clues or "flares" to the people they trust. These flares are subtle signs that there is something on their mind that they might like to talk about. You might hear, "Well, who knows if the chemo will work," or "I don't know if I'll even be here next summer."

You might bring up plans for Christmas and see your loved one look away or give a subtle shoulder shrug.

Be alert for flares.

It can be tempting to squash them as soon as you see them. "Don't say that!" you might respond, or "Of course you'll be here next summer."

These responses may be so automatic that you stomp out the flare before you even notice that it's there.

Try not to do this. Listen and watch for the subtle suggestion that your loved one is thinking about their mortality and wants to talk about it. What should you do if you notice a flare? You can say one of the most powerful phrases in the communication arsenal. You can say: "Tell me more about that."

Your goal is simply to make space for your loved one to share what is on their mind. It isn't yours to fix or figure out or control in any way. You are simply creating a container, a vessel, for your loved one's musings.

Your gift is to create space for their thoughts or questions or fears or impressions. Put your phone away, lean in, and truly hear them. You can use reflective listening if it feels right, but your primary approach can simply be, "Tell me more."

Sometimes your person may not want to share any more information, and that's fine too. You don't need to push them; you simply want to allow them to share more if they feel inclined to do so.

When you want to talk more than your loved one does

Sometimes your person may have no interest in talking about any of the stuff that you want to talk about. You may be poised and ready to use reflective listening and appropriate use of silence. You may have gathered the courage to talk about all the hard things, only to find that your loved one just wants to watch TV. Maybe you tried different approaches to get them to open up, but you get shut down every time. What can you do about this?

Nothing.

You may be convinced that it would be better to get it all out in the open and talk about all the hard things. I agree with you. And if I were your loved one, we'd have multi-hour conversations about life and death, meaning, purpose, and maybe even what we think will happen after we leave our beautiful blue planet. But your loved one isn't me.

When you and I are face-to-face with our own mortality, we can talk all night long if we want to. But this journey is your loved one's journey, and they get to make their own rules. So, if they don't want to talk, that's okay. Not the "fine, do it your way," kind of okay, but really, truly, and completely fine. You can check in occasionally, because they may feel more like sharing next week or next month, but be sure that you aren't badgering them. How can you know if you're badgering them? Just ask.

Self-Compassion

This stuff is hard.

Worrying that your loved one's health is declining or that they might die is heart-wrenching. Having to talk to them about it can seem like pouring hot sauce into your gaping heart-shaped wound.

You are doing the best that you can.

Don't let yourself be mean to yourself. You will avoid some conversations or wish you'd had them sooner. You will show up cranky or bossy, and sometimes your person will be grumpy or distant or impossible to reach. It's all okay. Just do the best that you can. Your best is good enough.

If you hear criticism coming your way from inside your mind, try to dodge out of its way. Then see if you can find a place of self-compassion. If your dearest friend were facing what you are facing, what would you say to that friend? I'll bet you'd be kind and empathetic and supportive. Your vibe would probably be something like, "You're doing your best," or, "This is really tough," or, "I'm here for you."

Can you find that kindness and compassion for yourself?

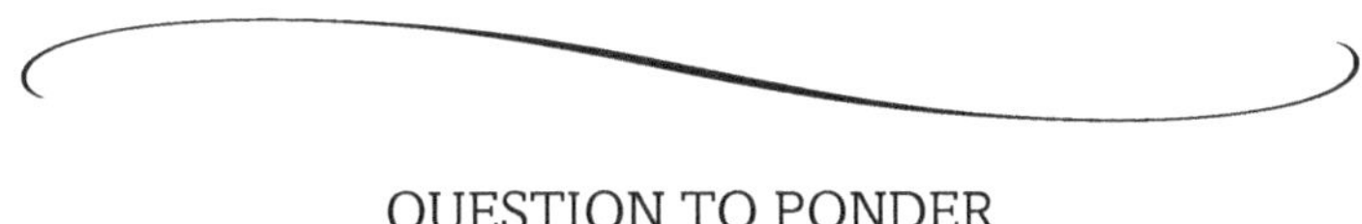

QUESTION TO PONDER

How have you been treating yourself? Could you be kinder, more compassionate, and more understanding towards yourself?

FAMILY DISCUSSION QUESTION

Are there any conversations that we have been avoiding?

EXERCISE

Approach a family member about a topic that you've been afraid to bring up.

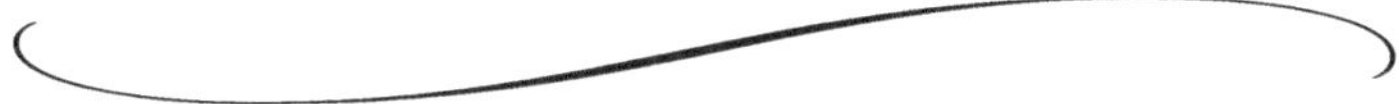

CHAPTER 13

Avoid Negative Positivity

Frank was a sixty-seven-year-old man who had been admitted to the hospital with abdominal pain. He'd been feeling sick for almost a month but had tried to tough it out, so he hadn't mentioned his bloating, abdominal pressure, or nausea to anyone, not even his wife.

Eventually, his wife noticed that Frank wasn't himself and she took him to the hospital. He protested the whole way.

After multiple blood tests and scans and many hours in the emergency department, Frank's doctors admitted him to the hospital. He found himself in a hospital bed with beeping machines and a blaring TV. His wife and three daughters were there too, sitting in uncomfortable silence.

Everyone looked up when I opened the door.

"Hi. I'm Doctor Chiaramonte," I said brightly. "I'm from the palliative medicine service. Is this an okay time to chat?"

Frank and his family were polite but distracted. They answered my questions, but they felt far away and hard to reach.

It turned out that the oncologist had been in to see them just before me and had dropped a bomb. Frank had advanced pancreatic cancer.

At one point I asked Frank if he had anything particular on his mind. He spoke softly, almost under his breath.

"What if the chemo doesn't work?"

It came out more like he was talking to himself, rather than asking me a question.

I was about to say, "Can you tell me more about what you're thinking?" which is my standard response when someone throws out a flare that they have something heavy on their mind.

But before I could get it out, Frank's wife and daughters shot up and hurled themselves towards his hospital bed.

"WHAT DID YOU SAY?" his wife shrieked.

"What if the chemo doesn't work?" Frank repeated, more clearly this time. "The doctor said it might not work."

The four women, who Frank loved most in the world, shot word daggers at him all at once.

"What did you say?! Don't you ever say that again!"

"Don't say that Daddy! Of course, it's going to work!"

"How can you say that?!? You'd better not say that!"

"Do *not* talk that way! Everything is going to be fine!"

I couldn't tell which words belonged to whom, but Frank got the message loud and clear. The message he received was, "Those thoughts are not welcome here."

Frank's wife brought her face close to his and shook her finger at him like he was a naughty child.

"You have to be positive!" she said in a shrill and bossy tone.

I knew that she was worried about Frank, but her energy was more critical than concerned.

Frank shrunk back into his hospital bed, deflated. He didn't say another word, and his wife and daughters, satisfied that there would be no more negativity, sat back down and turned towards the small wall-mounted TV.

What happened in Frank's room that day happens in hospital rooms, bedrooms, and living rooms every day, everywhere. Scary or uncomfortable ideas get squashed and smashed into boxes and locked tightly away so no one has to look at them. For a little while everyone in the room feels safer. The trouble is, locking scary ideas in metaphorical boxes doesn't make anyone safer; it just makes people lonely in their fear.

Frank's wife and daughters were trying to be helpful. They loved Frank. The idea that his cancer might not respond to the only thing offered to keep him alive was terrifying to them and they wanted to make the scary feelings stop. Most likely, this was not a conscious decision. They felt fear rising up and they collectively and unconsciously smashed it down. Unfortunately, this frantic whack-a-mole attempt to feel better doesn't work, and unconscious responses like this can leave families feeling distant and people with illness feeling abandoned.

Occasionally, denial is pursued as a family with eyes wide open, and this can be a reasonable temporary approach. Well-placed denial can be a balm that soothes the psyche. If everyone in the room agrees that there is "nothing to see here," denial can help to build resistance to the painful reality of an advancing illness. It doesn't work forever, but allowing the moments of painful awareness in slowly is fine if a tsunami of realization is too much to bear all at once. It is crucial, however, to assure that everyone in the family is intentionally digging their own head-sized hole in the sand. It is okay, for a while, if everyone in the family agrees to look away from the pain. If Frank had been on board with this approach, it would have been an acceptable temporary plan. But if someone in the family is a truth-teller, especially if it is the person with the illness, a family who refuses to take off their blinders can create unnecessary isolation and loneliness.

Frank was a truth-teller.

He didn't want to hide from what was happening. It was on his mind, and he wanted to talk about it. Frank didn't want to face the scary parts alone; he wanted to lean on his people for support. His wife and daughters were his people, but they had turned away from him and become unreachable.

When Frank asked, "What if the chemo doesn't work?" he wasn't really talking about the effectiveness of cancer drugs. He wasn't talking about cancer at all. Frank was using the words that he had to share a fear rising up within him. He was sharing the fear that he was going to die. Yet when Frank admitted out loud that the beast threatening his life might win the battle, his family responded from a place of fear rather than love.

When Frank's wife and daughters yelled, "Don't say that!" and "You have to be positive!" their heart was saying "I love you. I can't imagine life without you."

But what they communicated was more like, "We can't tolerate your fears. You'll have to handle them alone."

They weren't able to hold space for Frank's fears or help him to feel safe and supported in the face of his uncertain future. They communicated clearly, whether they intended to or not, that he was not to speak his fear out loud in their presence. They left Frank to wallow in that fear all by himself.

Frank's family didn't mean to shame him for being scared or emotionally abandon him, but that is exactly what they did.

This is a form of toxic positivity.

Toxic positivity isn't positive, but it is most certainly toxic.

It is a positively toxic way to make a person who is struggling with something feel worse after talking to you than they did when they were alone.

If you have ever heard phrases like these, then you've been a victim of toxic positivity:

"Don't be sad. Everything happens for a reason"

"Don't talk that way! You need to be positive."

"If you don't think positively, you'll never get better."

"You're strong! There's no need for you to be afraid."

The problem with toxic positivity is that it doesn't make us feel better. Our words aren't powerful enough to save us from sadness, fear, or grief, but they do have the power to hurt us.

"Don't talk that way."

"You don't mean that."

"You have to look on the bright side."

"Everything is going to be okay."

"God won't let you down. You just have to stay positive and believe."

Adult children say these things to their parents, wives say them to their husbands, and siblings say them to each other. Everyone wants everyone else to be positive. And the more dire the situation, the more aggressively the positivity police act up.

When a loving wife or friend or sister or child says something like this to someone who is ill, they are hoping to make things better. They are trying to will good things into being or boost up their loved one's mood. There is no doubt that all the "just be positive" talk comes from a loving heart. Unfortunately, it doesn't end up being a loving act.

When something crummy is going on, like a serious illness that is progressing or refuses to go away, well-meaning positivity can be toxic. Toxic positivity doesn't honor the depth of the pain that the person is experiencing or allow them to feel their anger or grief or sadness. It tries to whitewash the situation with happy words, but instead of clearing out the negative feelings it covers them up with a waterproof coating that makes them fester and stink. Imagine a wall covered in spreading black mold that a misguided homeowner covers in thick, white paint. It might look pretty for the moment, but under the shiny, smiling whitewash is some funky stuff that is going to find its way back out.

Evelyn was a vibrant woman in her fifties with a high lilting voice and elevated perfect eyebrows that made her look perpetually pleasantly surprised. She smiled through our entire first visit. Evelyn had recently received a diagnosis of stage IV gastric cancer. She was pursuing chemotherapy and had made an appointment to see me, at her oncologist's recommendation, because she was having difficulty sleeping.

"I just want you to know that I am doing fine!" she said.

In fact, this was the first thing that she said to me. I tend to match my patients' energy, especially when I'm just meeting someone, because it can help to build rapport, so I answered with, "That's great! Tell me more."

"I'm the positive one," she said. "I'm just a positive person. It's who I am. I've always been that way," she told me. "Everyone in my life knows that. People come to me when they need a lift."

Her words may have been positive, but her smile didn't reach her eyes. I could feel sadness seeping out from behind her happy mask.

I got the feeling that Evelyn was bound by positive, toxic handcuffs. Her identity was entirely intertwined with being 'the positive one.' Yet what is 'the positive one' supposed to do when she is told she has stage IV cancer? Does she still need to cheerlead everyone else in her life when they lose a job or have a fight with their spouse or need to put their dog to sleep? Evelyn needed support now, but no one had fired her from her position as chief positivity officer. Her identity as the community mood elevator has gone from being a gift that gave her joy to a burden that threated to smother and crush her.

She was valiantly trying to hang on to her sunshine and light identity, but it was getting harder. Her insides, which were scared and sad and overwhelmed, were no longer aligned with her outsides. But she was hanging on tightly to her old self, gritting her teeth into a forced perky smile. Evelyn couldn't imagine herself as anything but 'the positive one,' so not only did she have advanced cancer, but she was losing her identity, too. No wonder she couldn't sleep.

I gave some thought to how I should proceed. If being relentlessly positive was part of her coping mechanism, and if it was helping her, I certainly didn't want to dismantle it. Anything that helps someone cope in difficult times, as long as it isn't dangerous for them or someone else, is just fine. I got the impression, though, that this aggressively positive stance wasn't helping Evelyn; it was trapping her. It was drowning her. And it wasn't even clear if her family and friends were requiring this of her or if she was requiring it of herself.

I started with reflecting what she'd said to me.

"So, it sounds like everyone expects you to be the positive one," I said. "You have to be upbeat all the time, no matter what's going on. Did I get that right?"

"Yes! That's my superpower," she said proudly.

Hmmm. I didn't want to steal her superpower, but I did want to give her permission to take a vacation from being a superhero if she wanted that.

I started with, "I'll bet you've supported a lot of people."

"Oh yes, everyone comes to me!" she said.

"What a gift you are to your people," I said to her. I meant it. "I'm sure you've put a lot of good into this world."

"I hope so," she said, more softly now.

"It does sound a little exhausting, though," I said. "You always have to be the positive one and lift everyone else up. It makes me tired thinking about it."

I wanted her to know that she could be proud of herself for being a helper and also admit that she was tired.

She paused. Her posture softened and she blinked her eyes a few times. In a voice that was lower and slower she said, "Yeah. It does get tiring."

We sat in silence for a few minutes.

"But what am I supposed to do?" she asked me. "It's who I am."

She paused and shifted in her chair. This time she spoke softly, lowering her gaze to the floor.

"I just don't know if I can do it anymore."

This was an important moment. We sat in silence for a while to let that statement percolate and send its tendrils deep into her awareness. She was tired. And she wasn't sure that she could do it anymore. She wasn't sure that she could deal with stage IV cancer and also carry and lift the emotions of all the other people in her life.

I was proud of her for voicing her quandary; giving words to the paradox that she identified as a relentlessly positive person who didn't feel all that positive right now.

When people share statements like "I don't know if I can do this anymore," family members, friends, and even doctors often try to shut them down. It doesn't matter if they mean "I can't tolerate the chemotherapy anymore," or "I'm tired of making everyone else happy," or "I just can't care for mom all by myself." The urge is strong to say something like, "Oh, you can definitely do it. You're strong. I have faith in you."

Sometimes that is the right thing to say, and it can make people feel inspired and supported. Encouraging someone's strength when they are asking to be encouraged is a loving act with powerful potential. But when the exact same words are used to force someone's difficult, painful feelings underground, they can harm instead of help.

How can you know when positivity will be helpful and when it may be wounding? Simple. You ask. If someone you love says "I don't know if I can do this anymore," try responding with "tell me more about that," or "what do you mean when you say that?"

If they say "I'm doubting myself. I just need some inspiration," or "I need a boost," feel free to boost away. You can go all in with "you've got this!" or "I have faith in you," or "you're the strongest person I know." But if, instead, they say something like, "I'm getting tired," or "I think things might be changing," or "I think the treatment isn't working," I suggest a very different approach. In this case, reflective listening is the way to go. You could say something like, "It sounds like you're feeling exhausted," or "you're worried the treatment won't work?" Make space for your person to explore the nuances of their feelings and give them permission to get off the positivity train.

Helpful Positivity

Gratitude is all the rage. People have gratitude journals and gratitude groups and gratitude meditations and gratitude retreats.

I'm pro gratitude. Gratitude is good. Gratitude is noticing and appreciating the flowers.

However, when gratitude gets confused with toxic positivity it goes from being helpful and inspiring to feeling heavy and smothering. Evelyn felt smothered. Yet because she confused toxic positivity with healthy positivity and gratitude, she struggled to free herself from that unpleasant and unhelpful weight.

I asked Evelyn to share what she didn't like about what was happening. She hesitated at first, but once she got going a whole lot of backed up junk came pouring out. I was proud of her! She told me about how much she hated chemo, that being nauseous sucked, that she was afraid her husband would leave her now that she was bald, and that she missed who she used to be. After she ran out of negative things to talk about, she laughed.

"You're right. I do feel better!"

Her energy was different. Lifted. Her face was more open, her eyes sparkled, and her movements were fluid. She was, simply, lighter.

Once she lanced the abscess of 'cancer sucks' pus that she had covered over with a sparkly band-aid, she felt relieved. She acknowledged all of the poop that she was facing and was now ready to look for the flowers.

I suggested that she fill in the blanks of the following sentence:

"I really don't like ______________, but at least ______________."

She started with "I really don't like that I have cancer, but at least I have a supportive family."

"Great job," I said. "Do it again."

"I really don't like that I'm bald, but at least my head isn't too lumpy."

We laughed at that one.

"Do it again."

"I really don't like that I'm so tired, but at least I'm catching up on books that I've been meaning to read."

I asked her to do one where the two ideas weren't related.

She said, "I hate chemotherapy but at least I have air conditioning."

"Excellent job!" I told her. "This is helpful positivity. It acknowledges the hard stuff, then shifts your gaze to something lighter and more pleasant. Sometimes you can even find something beautiful."

You can do this all day long. In fact, I recommend that you do just that.

"I don't like that it's raining, but at least I got a good parking spot."

"I don't like that my house is messy, but at least my fridge is full."

"I don't like that my dog pees in the house, but at least she is adorable and cuddles with me on the couch."

Don't forget to do some that are unrelated. "I don't like that my boss is so critical but at least my tomatoes are growing well this year."

This exercise is a skill builder for gratitude. The more you do it, the more you'll continue to do it. Over time it becomes easier and more automatic. Once you add this practice into your day, you'll find that almost every time you complain about something you will automatically find an "at least."

This year we had to cut down the huge, ailing maple tree in my backyard. I had been talking to that tree almost daily for twenty years. She felt like my backyard best friend or big sister. We had watched the children grow up together, and I had thoroughly anthropomorphized that tree. Watching her get dismantled limb by limb hurt my heart. I made myself watch the brutal process and then sobbed until all that was left of my old friend was a stump.

I was heartbroken.

Somehow, watching her dismemberment, from a mighty and towering queen to a pile of debris, felt tragic. Maybe it was because my children had recently left for college, and it was the end of an era of playing with them under her loving canopy. Maybe it foreshadowed my own mortality. I just know that it made me sad.

We kept a slice of her massive trunk that we thought we might use as a coffee table, but mostly so I could keep a piece of her nearby. But when we rolled the massive piece of wood onto its side, we discovered something totally unexpected. A large portion of the trunk was so soft inside that I could scoop it out with a small stick. That tree, my friend with her huge, heavy branches that could have killed me or those that I love if they had fallen on us, had been rotting from the inside out. Her monstrous limbs were being held in the air by sawdust. I was flooded with gratitude that we had taken her down before she had inadvertently hurt, or even killed, one of us.

Here's my "I hate______ but at least______" statement:

"I hate that we had to take down our beloved tree, but at least we had twenty years together and we took her down before one of her branches fell on us."

This ability to positively reframe an unpleasant, painful, unfair, or generally yucky situation becomes life-changing over time. It is helpful for both the toxic negativity and the toxic positivity set, because it acknowledges both states—there is poop, but there are also flowers.

Sometimes even literal flowers. Our lawn had a big scar where the tree had been and we planted a bunch of annuals there, imagining that seeing flowers where our tree friend used to be would make us happy. Repeatedly, the flowers would start to grow and then disappear. Then the plants themselves started getting smaller instead of bigger. We couldn't figure out what was going on. That is, until I started working from my screened porch that looks onto the yard. One day, as I sat quietly typing on my laptop, I noticed a momma bunny and her adorable baby hopping into my flower garden and helping themselves to the tasty buds and leaves. Mystery solved. Even though they were destroying what I had spent money and time creating, I was struck by the sweetness of a momma finding something yummy to nourish her baby.

"I don't like that my lawn looks kind of ugly and my flowers are all gone, but at least that momma bunny is able to feed her baby and I get to watch them, which makes me feel happy."

After the tree was gone, I was chatting with my neighbor over our backyard fence. I was bemoaning the loss of the tree and she said:

"There are worse things than losing a tree. I have a bad cancer, you know."

Oh goodness. I hadn't known. Her story put my tree drama right back where it belonged. My issue was an inconvenience while hers was life changing. Yet despite her struggles she instinctively used the "I don't like/but at least" method. Her next statement offered a realistically positive perspective on the challenges that she was facing.

"I'm getting chemo," she shared, "but I'm tolerating it okay."

The more you practice this, the easier and more automatic it becomes. It makes sweet times even sweeter and hard times a little easier to bear.

Can you think of one or two "I don't like/but at least" situations in your own life?

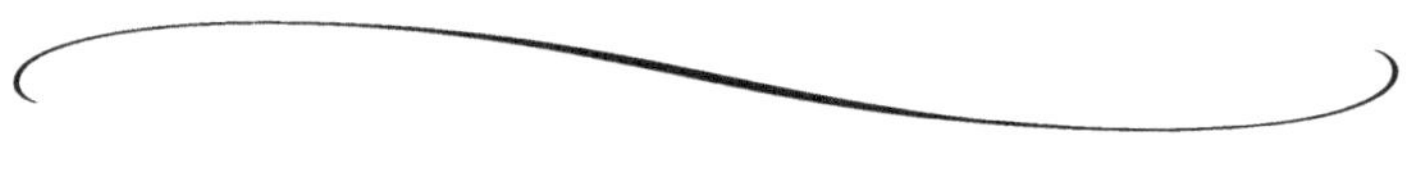

QUESTION TO PONDER

Where does toxic positivity show up in your life?

FAMILY DISCUSSION QUESTION

Do we allow each other to express scary or uncomfortable ideas?

EXERCISE

Practice, "I don't like ______, but at least ______."
Try to do it at least three times a day.

CHAPTER 14

Flirt with Forgiveness

"This patient doesn't have any family," the hospital physician said. "And he can't make any medical decisions for himself. Can you see him and help us figure out what to do?"

"Hi Mr. P," I said when I entered his hospital room.

He looked up at me and smiled a huge, friendly smile. I smiled back and took a seat by his bedside. "I'm Dr. Chiaramonte and I'm happy to meet you."

"You can call me Paul," he said, and he reached out to shake my hand.

His handshake was firm, and I could tell that he used to be a powerful man. I had a feeling that he had lived a hard life, and he had clearly declined since his vital years. He was frail and thin, and his gnarled, overgrown toenails were a giveaway that things hadn't been going well at home.

Paul was seventy-three years old, and he had just had a stroke.

His face drooped on one side and his opposite arm and leg weren't moving. Although he knew his name, he couldn't tell me where he was or why he wasn't at home. He didn't know his address or who the president was, and he knew the month but not the year. He didn't remember how he'd gotten to the hospital, although he did tell me that he didn't like the food.

Paul was confused. I'd never met him before, but since he had lived alone prior to the stroke, I imagined that this level of confusion was new. Yet when I asked Paul if he had any children, he gave such a clear and specific answer that I believed him.

"I have a son . . . but he's in jail," Paul told me. "I wasn't a very good father, and I didn't teach him right," he added.

"Tell me more about your son," I said.

Paul told me what a good boy his son, Brian, had been and he expressed regret that he'd missed a lot of Brian's childhood. Paul had broken up with Brian's mother when their child was little, and his visits over the years had been inconsistent.

"It's probably my fault that he's in prison," he said.

Paul didn't have a spouse or domestic partner, and Brian was his only child. Paul's parents were no longer living, and his only brother had also died. The medical team was looking for a family member who could help make decisions for Paul and help them make a plan for him. He clearly couldn't live alone anymore, and no one was sure what to do.

Paul asked us to try to contact his son.

"He might not want to talk to me," Paul told me. "I wasn't a good father." He was quiet for a moment before he added, "I wouldn't blame him, but I want to tell him that I'm sorry."

The medical team had incorrectly assumed that we wouldn't be able to reach Brian in prison, so they hadn't even tried. But our palliative care social worker found him, got permission to talk to him, and got him on the phone.

Brian had some feelings.

"My dad is an a**hole," Brian said loudly. "Why would I want to help him out now?"

The social worker shared with Brian that his dad had asked us to contact him, and she made it clear that Paul knew that Brian might not be interested in talking to us, or to him. She told Brian that his dad had shared that he wasn't a great dad and that he wanted to tell Brian that he was sorry.

Brian said he'd think about it and asked us to contact him again in a couple of days.

The next time our team contacted Brian, his tone was softer. He'd been thinking about his dad, he told us, and he wanted to talk to him. The social worker worked her magic with the prison administrators and made it happen.

I don't know how deep a conversation they had, given Paul's limitations, but I know that something important happened. Suddenly Paul had family. The medical team gave Brian updates on how his dad was doing, and they relied on him to make medical decisions when Paul couldn't do that for himself. Clearly, some sort of healing had happened, and I imagine that this soothed painful wounds for both of them.

I found it ironic that it was Paul's stroke, certainly an unwelcome event, that had reconnected him with the son that he had been pining for and thought he would never speak to again.

It doesn't always work this way.

One of my other patients, Max, had an advanced prostate cancer and his treatments weren't working. He talked openly about the fact that he would likely die from this cancer, and he wanted to focus on enjoying whatever time he had. He still felt well so he planned to travel and eat delicious food and surround himself with the music that had soothed his soul throughout his life.

When I was getting to know him, I asked, "Do you have any children?"

Yikes. The air in the room got instantly chilly. His face got pinched and he puffed out his chest. "No. I do not have any children," he answered slowly and deliberately.

He stared at me with steely eyes when he said it. I did not know what to make of his response, but I got the message that I had poked the bear.

Over time, it came out that he had a grown daughter and son, from whom he was completely estranged. As he got sicker, we asked multiple times if he wanted us to contact them and his answer never wavered, "Absolutely not."

This story doesn't tie up nicely with a bow. There is no happy family reunion ending. I share it because it goes that way sometimes. Sometimes illness spurs estranged families to find their way back to each other, and sometimes it doesn't.

You might even find yourself caring for a parent, or other person, with whom you've had a difficult relationship. Maybe they've hurt you, emotionally, physically, or sexually. Maybe you've been caring for them, one way or another, for your entire life. Maybe they just popped back into your life because they need something from you. Maybe you simply don't like them.

Families are complicated.

You may even be estranged from a family member, as I am, and have to choose whether or not you will participate in their care. There is no one right approach.

Yet flirting with forgiveness works no matter which story you find yourself in. You can flirt with forgiving your loved one or you can flirt with forgiving yourself. You can flirt with forgiving your siblings, the doctors, your childhood nanny, your parents, your spouse, your drooling dog, the Universe, or your God.

But you only have to flirt with forgiveness, you don't have to go all in.

⁓

Forgiveness talk can have a toxic positivity flavor if you aren't careful.

"You have to forgive her," you might hear. "She's dying."

There's an unsaid but clearly communicated second part to that sentence, which is something like, "What's wrong with you?"

Encouraging someone to forgive can feel like an expectation with a pinch of judgment.

But here's the thing: we don't walk in each other's shoes, and forgiveness can't be mandated. If someone has wronged you in some way, it might be hard to forgive them, and getting cancer or some equally rough disease does not absolve them of their sins. If you are able to fully forgive them, that's terrific. Forgiveness is definitely lighter than holding on to pain and it is a worthwhile goal that is worth the cost of a therapist. But lifting the burden of old hurts is a marathon, not a sprint. It does not magically lift when a doctor says "you have cancer" or when the end of someone's life is in view.

So, my oddly conflicting message to you is this: forgive your people if you can, but don't worry if you can't. And if you don't even want to try, that's okay too.

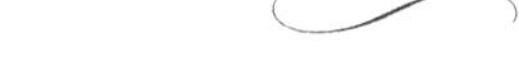

You Can Always Forgive Yourself

You've probably done a lot of things wrong. You've broken promises and hearts and maybe a fancy vase or expensive lamp. You've made embarrassing mistakes, told a bunch of white lies and likely a few hurtful ones too. Maybe you've stolen something or hurt someone's feelings. Maybe you've spoken harshly to people that you care about or forgotten to say happy birthday. You've probably yelled at your kids and left the dog home alone for too many hours. You may have messed up at work or made copies of your naked butt on the office copier. I don't know what you've done, but I'll bet you have stories.

Making Amends

Forgiving yourself is complicated.

On the one hand you are a beautiful and precious child of the Universe, and you deserve unconditional love and acceptance. On the other hand, you might have had some jackass moments that you really should apologize for. Forgiving yourself for bad behavior without making amends has a narcissistic flavor to it, and that's not what we're going for.

Some radical self-reflection is in order. Settle yourself in a comfy chair and take stock. Is there something that you should apologize for? Someone with whom you should reconnect? Do you have amends to make? If so, that's terrific. No judgment. You're human and we all falter. It's fine. If there is something that you have a feeling you should do or say, go ahead and make a plan to do it or say it.

Now that you've self-reflected and made plans to make amends, it is time to forgive yourself. Forgive yourself for all the times that you've been an imperfect person, said imperfect words, or done imperfect things. Your behaviors may have been imperfect, but your essence, the you that is underneath your mask or your shell, is always worthy of love, acceptance, and forgiveness.

This is easy to say, but for some people it is hard to do. If you tend to be hard on yourself or have sky high expectations, you may have a long list of your failures and shortcomings in your metaphorical back pocket. If you are struggling more with forgiving someone else, hang tight, we'll be getting to that next. But there's something that I'd like you to consider. Sometimes it can be easier to feel anger or frustration at someone else than to feel our own shame or guilt. Yet for other people it can feel easier to blame ourselves than to honestly review how people we love have failed or wronged us. Most often, there's a little of this and a little of that. So, I encourage you to explore both sides of the forgiveness coin. Is there a way for you to forgive yourself and also to forgive the other people in your life?

How to Forgive Yourself

It's easy for me to say that you should forgive yourself for all the times that you've messed up or all the ways that you are imperfect. I struggle with this myself, so I know it isn't easy. Taking specific action works much better than simply proclaiming that all is well, but what works for me might annoy the heck out of you. Here are some self-forgiveness actions to consider:

1. **Focus on What You Learned from the Experience**

Difficult experiences are often growth generators. You are more likely to find your surprising strength, achieve a new perspective, or uncover a unique passion after a challenging experience than after a day running errands or folding the laundry. I refer to an experience that is rough but growth-inducing as an AFGO (Another F-ing Growth Opportunity). If you didn't like how you behaved with your loved one, but it was an AFGO, spend some time ruminating on the learning and the growth.

2. **Practice Self-Compassion**

You've already heard about self-compassion, but it's so important and so underused that it deserves another mention. The practice of self-compassion involves actively and intentionally talking to yourself the way that you would talk to someone who is very dear to you. If your very best friend in the world were cranky with her aging mother or decided that her dad really needs to move to a memory care facility, what would you say to her? Would you tell her that she is ungrateful and selfish? Would you beat her up and make her feel small? I hope not. You'd probably say things like, "You've done the very best that you could," or "This is really hard."

Speaking to yourself in this way, with kindness and understanding, is most of the way to self-forgiveness.

3. Practice Letting Go Rituals

Your perceived shortcomings may be sticky. Even if you have jumped on the self-forgiveness train, your brain may have all kinds of "Yeah, but . . ." stories to remind you why you shouldn't forgive yourself just yet. Physical letting go rituals can help. There are unlimited options, but some of my favorites are:

- Write down your perceived shortcomings on paper, paint over the words with pretty colors, cut up the painted paper, and create a collage. I like the symbolism of turning tough stuff into beautiful stuff.
- Write down what you feel shame or guilt about and burn the paper in the fireplace. Imagine your mistakes floating up in the smoke and disappearing.
- Find a stream or other running water. Choose a leaf and speak your perceived offenses out loud. Imagine placing them on the leaf and watch them float away.
- Use your breath. Imagine breathing in a healing light and breathing out any negativity, guilt, or shame. Imagine the heavy energy floating away from your body. Notice that the more negativity you blow away, and healing light you invite in, the lighter and more joyful you feel.

4. Use Guided Imagery

Guided imagery is an easy way to calm your sympathetic nervous system, which is the part of the nervous system responsible for the stress response. It involves listening to someone, often through a recording, who guides you to imagine relaxing or health-inducing scenes. In addition to encouraging relaxation, it may encourage your mind to see the world through a more connected and forgiving lens. Any relaxing guided imagery can be helpful, but you might find that a particular type of meditation called a "LovingKindness" meditation is especially helpful for self-forgiveness. You can find a sample "LovingKindness" meditation at www.CopingSupport.com.

5. Read Books About Self-Forgiveness

There are many wonderful books about self-forgiveness. It can be helpful to explore the concept more fully with a great book and a warm cup of tea or coffee, enjoyed in a cozy chair. If you'd like a suggested book list, you can find one at www.CopingSupport.com.

6. Write Yourself a Self-Compassion Letter

Start this letter "Dear (you) . . ." Write from the heart and outline all the amazing things about you. Describe how you've helped the world, the ways in which you are kind, your personal strengths, and the things that people who like you say behind your back. Imagine how your dearest friend would describe you. Once you write the letter, put it away for a few days then read it out loud to yourself.

7. Make an Offering

If self-forgiveness feels especially out of reach, making an 'offering' may help. You can light a candle, do something kind for another person, or donate money to a cause that is close to your heart.

8. Have a Ceremony

Sometimes you just need a ceremony. Ceremonies help us deal with the important moments of life: the hard ones, the happy ones, and the milestones. You could have a forgiveness ceremony, a 'cleansing' ceremony, a self-compassion ceremony, a chocolate ice-cream ceremony or any other ceremony that feels right.

9. Talk to a Therapist

Therapists are great. Sometimes just talking it out and having your experiences mirrored by another person can make space for new insights and growth.

10. Explore Journaling

If you prefer to be your own therapist, a journal is a powerful tool. Whether you're sharing your thoughts in a beautiful notebook or typing into your laptop, getting your thoughts out of your head can give you a new perspective on the situation.

11. Explore Healing Modalities

There are many healers who can help you let go of sticky thoughts and self-criticism and open you up to self-compassion and well-being. You might consider trying acupuncture, Emotional Freedom Technique (EFT)/Tapping, Reiki, somatic experiencing, and others. Try out as many different healing modalities as you can. This is an experiment to identify what you should do more of.

12. Use a Self-Forgiveness Mantra

The words that you say to yourself have the power to impact how you feel. If your words are unsupportive and unkind, you will feel unsupported and hurt. A self-forgiveness mantra can be used to replace your negative self-talk with a clear and forgiving message. You might say your mantra to yourself ten times while you brush your teeth. Or five times before you eat. Or twenty times before you go to sleep. Or all three. It can be helpful to hook the mantra to something that you're already doing so you don't forget to do it. See below for a list of self-forgiveness mantras.

Self-Forgiveness Mantras

- I am a good person
- I forgive myself for being imperfect
- I am worthy of forgiveness
- Sometimes I make mistakes and that's okay because everyone makes mistakes
- I learn from my mistakes
- I forgive others so I can forgive myself
- I deserve kindness and compassion
- I am good enough just as I am
- I am kind and wise
- Making mistakes helps me grow
- Forgiveness is strength
- I forgive myself

Forgiving Other People

People are imperfect. Put more bluntly, sometimes people suck. Even the nicest people may hurt your feelings, fail to show up for you like you think they should, or get cranky just when you were hoping they'd be supportive. Some people don't need much forgiving, but others need a ton.

Feelings can be complicated when someone that you love is ill. You may feel empathy for them because they are sick, and you wish with all of your being that they were well. Yet if they have wounded you in the past, been a lousy parent or bossy sibling, or if your relationship has been hot and cold over the years, it can be hard to make space for all the conflicting feelings as your loved one's health declines.

This is normal.

One of my favorite phrases is: "Don't judge your insides by other people's outsides."

It works perfectly here. The over-the-top expressions of love that you see on social media or in prayer email chains when someone is ill can make it look like other people's families are overflowing with pure and uncomplicated love and affection. Don't be fooled. As a physician, I have seen the dark underbelly of many families. Trust me, if the emotions in your family are complex, you are not alone.

Just because you fear losing your loved one, or painfully watching them decline, that doesn't mean that the old wounds magically disappear. They might, and if that happens a happy dance is in order. Sometimes being faced with the loss of someone you love erases all their past offenses. But sometimes it doesn't, and that's okay too.

Do you have to forgive your loved one?

No.

If forgiving your loved one is not in the cards, go back to the previous section and practice forgiving yourself for not forgiving your loved one. This doesn't in any way mean that you are doing something wrong by not forgiving them. Rather, it acknowledges that societal expectations of forgiving an ailing loved one are strong, so practicing self-forgiveness may be protective against current or future self-criticism.

Also, be sure not to treat forgiveness like a transaction. As in, "I'll forgive you and then you'll forgive me, and we'll live happily ever after." It doesn't always work that way. Sometimes, like for Paul and Brian, one person's forgiveness brings everyone back together, but often it isn't that simple. There may be layers of hurt feelings that peel back slowly, like an onion, and your forgiveness may not be enough to soothe all the hurt.

Your decision to act in a forgiving way is for *you*. It is not for anyone else, and it is not to heal all the family wounds. I hope that your decision to forgive brings healing to your family. I truly do. But I am certain that your decision to forgive will bring healing to you.

Forgiving Someone for Changing

One kind of forgiveness that you may not have thought about is forgiving someone for not being who they used to be. Hear me out. I know that you are not blaming your loved one for being sick, and you are likely being a dutiful friend or relative and helping as much as you feel able to. But it is a normal human response to be upset when someone that we care about is no longer the person that we once knew. Maybe your parent is now more like your child, or your spouse is no longer the leader of the household. Maybe you're used to being cared for and now you have to do all of the caring. Maybe you were planning to grow old with someone, and that is looking less and less likely. It is normal and okay to feel upset or even angry that life as you knew it has gotten all messed up. You can forgive yourself for feeling angry and you can forgive your person for not being who they used to be.

Flirting with Forgiving Someone Who Has Wronged You

If someone has fundamentally wronged you, fully forgiving them is a pretty high bar. You might need to invest in a few years of therapy or join your meditation teacher at the top of a mountain to achieve this milestone. These are worthwhile pursuits and I'm all for them. But for now, let's just start by flirting with forgiveness.

Many of the tools listed for forgiving yourself can be repurposed as you practice forgiving someone else. If you have a person in mind who needs forgiving, take a look at the list above to see which approaches appeal to you. Here are a few more that are specifically targeted to healing from hurtful experiences:

- **Identify the Hurt**

  You can't heal what you don't see. If you are stuffing your hurt deep underground and smiling through gritted teeth, it will be awfully hard to heal. This approach can make you withdraw and hide or lash out with anger or snarky sarcasm. Shining a bright light on the hurt that you've experienced, and the feelings that are rising up, is crucial for letting go and making space for forgiveness.

- **Consider Trying to Understand or Empathize with the Person Who Wronged You**

If this idea triggers or wounds you, feel free to skip this paragraph. Every situation is different and if you have been seriously hurt by someone, you may not be in a place to empathize with them. That's okay. But if understanding and empathy feels achievable, see if you can make space to understand what may have driven your person to treat you as they did. Write a list of what they have experienced over their lifetime, what they might have been feeling, what their fears or worries are, how they were parented, what they might be feeling now, and anything else that helps you understand and empathize with the imperfect person that they are.

- **Recall a Time When You Were Forgiven**

We all mess up sometimes, and it feels great to be forgiven. Tapping into that feeling of gratitude for forgiveness may help connect you with your forgiving self.

- **Write a Letter of Forgiveness**

Write a letter to your person, forgiving them for their foibles or shortcomings or hurtful behavior. Pour your heart into this letter. You may choose to read the letter out loud to your loved one, but only if you think it will be well received. If not, you can read the letter out loud to a trusted friend or family member. If that feels scary, you can read it out loud to yourself or to your cat, dog, or bearded dragon.

- **Create Something**

There is something about knitting a blanket, creating a collage, or planting a forgiveness garden that taps into our more connected and creative self. Play around with your playful self. The point is not to create a perfect final product, but to explore the part of you that connects with beauty, growth, and meaning. Use your creation to help you let go of the things that don't matter all that much.

- **Commemorate Your Forgiveness**
You might light a candle, say a prayer, gather a group of friends, or have a drumming circle to commemorate your efforts to forgive your loved one. It doesn't matter if you're just flirting with forgiveness. You've taken a step, and that deserves a party.

There will be times when you are blown away by your impressively generous and forgiving heart. Enjoy those times, because there will also be times when you feel pinched and contracted and you can't remember why you thought forgiveness was a good idea, anyway. Just ride the wave. Think of forgiveness as an action, not a feeling. You can practice forgiveness, even as your feelings come and go.

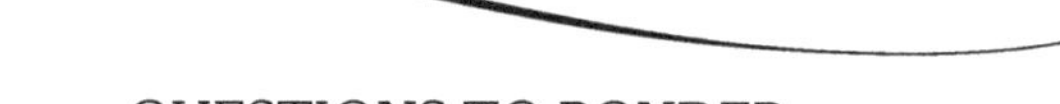

QUESTIONS TO PONDER

What can I forgive myself for? Who else do I want to forgive?

FAMILY DISCUSSION QUESTION

What can we forgive each other for?

EXERCISE

Create a plan to forgive yourself and/or someone in your life.

CHAPTER 15

Leave a Legacy

"I did what you suggested," Betty said, "and I'm *so* excited about it."

"Oooh, I can't wait to hear more," I said as I sat down next to her in the exam room.

Betty had an advanced cancer and, even though she was still getting immunotherapy, she realized that her time might be getting short. She had already had several different treatments that worked . . . until they didn't. At first, Betty thought there would always be another option, another helpful treatment to try, but recently her doctors had told her that this was their last shot. They discussed experimental treatments, but she wasn't interested in that. Her plan was to ride this treatment wave for as long as it worked and squeeze all the yummy juice out of life that she could.

She felt generally well, so during our last visit I had offered a suggestion.

"You know, since you feel so well . . . ," I said, "you could consider creating a legacy project of some sort. Sometimes I call them 'love projects.'"

She raised her eyebrows, interested but unsure.

"You don't have to do this, of course," I continued, "but some people choose to create something to leave as a legacy or a demonstration of love for their family or friends. It could be specifically for people you care about, or it could be just for you. And of course, if you live for a very long time, which I hope that you do, you haven't lost anything, you've just made a really nice gift for someone."

She was interested. "Okay, what do I do?"

"Well, that depends on what speaks to you," I said. "You could write a book or record the stories of your life. You could create a quilt or a painting for someone you love. You could make scrapbooks. You could write poems or letters to all your important people. You could write down your advice or wisdom for future generations to read. There are no rules."

"I like this," she said with excitement in her voice. "I like this."

"If the whole idea speaks to you," I said, "you could spend some time thinking about what a legacy or love project would look like for you."

When Betty came back to see me the next month, she was excited.

She had not only figured out a plan, but she had already completed it. She brought pictures.

"I decided that I wanted my grandchildren to know me and to know that I knew them," she said. "So, I made boxes."

"Boxes?" I raised my eyebrows.

"Boxes," she said. "Look."

Betty's boxes were beautiful. She had lovingly created eight different boxes, one for each of her eight precious grandchildren. The boxes were stunning on the outside, decorated to match the style and interests of each child, but the real gems were on the inside. In each box she had placed mementos that represented something that she appreciated about that child or something that they had done together. Some boxes had theater ticket stubs, others had dried flowers or pictures of her vegetable garden. Some had rocks or shells, some had sand from the beach. Each box had a picture of Betty with her grandchild and a special letter written from her heart to theirs.

"I'm still praying for a miracle," Betty told me. "If this treatment works, each kid can have their box when they turn eighteen."

I loved Betty's boxes.

When I think about why it is so important to have honest conversations early in the course of a serious illness, I think of Betty's boxes. Betty's pain was controlled, and her energy was good. She wanted to live more than anything in the world, but she was also willing to face whatever was coming with her eyes wide open. If Betty had been unwilling to acknowledge her prognosis and had waited until she was close to the end of her life to acknowledge that the end might be coming, she wouldn't have had the energy to create these beautiful, heartfelt boxes. Creating them didn't make her sad, it made her happy. She created those boxes from deep and joyful love, and making them didn't dim her hope one bit. They made her feel closer to her grandchildren and the process of creating them had been powerful and meaningful for Betty.

Not everyone makes boxes.

I've had other patients who asked their children to record interviews with them about their life or who have written short stories about their experiences. One of my patients was a painter, and she created personalized paintings for all her family members. Another was a graphic artist who created meaningful pieces for the people who had helped him on his life's journey. His gift to me hangs in my office and I think of him whenever I look at it. Some have shared their wisdom and advice in journals and others have used prepared prompts to answer questions about their lives. One of my patients made a video with instructions to play it at his funeral. He showed it to me, and it was hilarious. He wanted to be remembered as the funny guy that he had been for his entire life.

Not everyone wants to do a physical legacy or love project, and that's perfectly fine.

I knew that my patient, Maryanne, was a writer and an editor, so I thought her legacy project for her adult sons might involve something like writing them poetic and heartfelt letters or creating a personalized short story. She initially thought that would be her plan, too. But every time she came to see me, she sheepishly shared that she hadn't started them yet.

"You don't need to do this at all," I reassured her. "The idea doesn't speak to everyone and that's perfectly fine."

"No, no," she said. "It totally speaks to me; I just can't get started and I don't know why."

"The two things to think about," I told her, "Are *why* do you want to create a legacy project and *how* will you do it?"

"Well . . . ," she said slowly. "My *why* is that I want my boys to know how much I adore them. And I want them to feel connected to me."

"Okay, great," I said. "What would help your boys know that you adore them and feel connected to you?"

"Oh, wow," she said. "I just realized why I haven't been able to get started. My boys aren't big readers so I don't think I would really touch them with words. Plus, since I'm an editor, I'm always critiquing other people's writing. This is so important that I'm afraid I wouldn't quite hit the mark if I tried to put all my feelings into words."

"Wow. That's a powerful insight," I told her.

She seemed suddenly energetic and excited. "Oh, I know exactly what I'll do."

"Tell me." I felt excited too.

"I'm going to plan a trip," she said. "A special trip with each of them. Then we can make memories and take pictures and they can *feel* my love instead of reading about it. I'm going to start planning tonight."

And that's exactly what she did.

No one should create a legacy or love project because they feel pressured to do it. Or because they think that they *should* want to do it. Ideally, a legacy project bubbles up from deep inside begging to be released. It could be an object or an experience or a conversation. It might be big or small, take weeks or months to complete, or be over in a moment. A well-timed, open-hearted hug can be a legacy all by itself.

There are varied reasons why a person might choose to create a legacy project. Here are few examples:

To Show Love

This is a common motivation for starting a legacy project. I have created multiple things for my daughters because I want them to have physical manifestations of my love when I'm no longer here to provide that love to them directly. If your goal is to show love to someone dear to you, the quality of the product doesn't matter much at all. This is truly an 'it's the thought that counts' situation. If you dedicate your precious time and energy to crochet me a blanket, I don't care one bit if you drop some stitches. So, if love is your motivator, don't get too hung up on the details. Don't let the perfect be the enemy of the good.

To Provide Comfort

When my first daughter left for college, I was tear-stained and unsettled for longer than I expected. Perhaps because my own childhood was unhappy, I had embraced motherhood with my whole heart. So, when the youngest got ready to go, she knew that I would struggle with my newly-empty nest. I was brave through the packing of the car, the driving, the unpacking, and even the tight hug goodbye. It was when I walked back into our empty house that I fell apart. I went upstairs to my bedroom, planning to hide in bed and cry. When I walked into the room, I saw a teddy bear on my bed that I'd never seen before. There was a note that said, "Squeeze my paw."

I squeezed his paw and heard my sweet girl's voice. "Hi Mama . . ."

She had gone to Build-A-Bear™ and made a bear for me with a message in her voice. I was so touched that she had made this effort, and it truly did comfort me to hear her. I still squeeze that paw sometimes.

There are so many ways to bring comfort. A voice recording, photo blanket, personalized poem, heartfelt letter, handprint, scrapbook . . . There are endless options. If the goal is to bring comfort, thinking about the person who will receive the gift is helpful. I think my daughter realized that our house would be quiet once she was gone, and she knew I'd miss her voice.

To Give Future Advice

We parents love to give advice to our kids. We teach them how to brush their teeth, how to ride a bike, and how to be a good friend. We teach them how to stay safe when dating, how to get out of a toxic friendship, and how to drive in the snow. I haven't yet gotten the chance to teach my daughters about how to manage conflict in a long-term relationship, or that it's okay to feel overwhelmed when you first have a baby. I hope to be able to give that advice in person one day. If it looks like I won't get that chance, I plan to write down my advice so they can pull it out at the right time if they choose to.

Some people write their advice in a journal or a letter, while others record guidance in their own voice. Topics are unlimited but could include parenting, dating, traveling, running the household, and anything else that feels meaningful or important.

To Share Knowledge

You, your loved ones, and everyone that you know have gathered heaps of knowledge while walking through this life. We all know different stuff, but all of it is important and it's all useful to someone. So, whether you and your loved one know how to make birdhouses, keep a clean house, play chess, or take stunning photographs, sharing your knowledge, wisdom, and skill with the world is important and meaningful.

Writing articles, creating a recipe file, writing a how-to book, and recording educational videos are examples of ways to share knowledge with the world. I suppose this book is a legacy project for me.

To Share Experiences

Knowledge isn't the only thing worth sharing. Experiences are powerful, and it can be highly meaningful to share our experiences with the people that we love. We can share stories, pictures, or mementos of work, travel, relationships, creativity, spiritual life, parenting, connection with animals, cooking, and all the other things that make up a fully lived life.

To Make a Mark on The World

When my patient, Addie, got ovarian cancer, she worked almost as hard on her legacy project as she did on her treatment. She was a powerful fundraiser and networker, and she raised a ton of money for ovarian cancer research. She wanted to do all that she could to turn her difficult experience into something positive for the women who would sit in those chemo chairs long after she had. Fundraising is one way to make a mark on the world, but there are unlimited other possibilities.

Options include starting a scholarship, donating antiques to a museum, leaving money to an animal shelter, teaching an adult to read, or writing a book. Even smaller projects, like cataloguing the species of birds that visit a neighborhood bird feeder, can be meaningful.

To Make Life Easier for Others

My husband and I compiled a notebook labeled "Things You Will Need When We Die." We don't want our kids to have to unravel our finances when they are facing the loss of their parents. We both hope to live long lives, but in case the unthinkable happens, we have done what we can to avoid adding unneeded stress to our girls' deep grief.

To Leave Something Behind

My dad sculpts in marble. He travels every year to Tuscany to sculpt in Carrera marble, just like Michelangelo did. Many of his sculptures are ten feet tall, but I have two of the smaller ones in my back yard. After years of being outside, with the wind and the dirt and the birds, they aren't gleaming white anymore, but I am moved by them nearly every time I see them. They are heavy and robust, and they are in-your-face proof that my dad has spent time here on Earth.

The wish to leave something of ourselves behind after we're gone is a deep human desire. We can leave behind sculptures, but also woodwork, photographs, poetry, music, journals, quilts, knit sweaters, sewn creations, curated collections, and so much more.

What If Your Loved One Can't Do a Legacy Project?

Your loved one may be too sick or too tired to work on a legacy project. They may have advanced dementia and be unable to meaningfully contribute, but that doesn't mean that you're left out of this process.

If your person has lost the ability to create a project on their own, you or your family can take control of the wheel. Depending on the state of your loved one's body and mind, they may participate a lot, a little, or not at all. All those options are perfectly fine.

Check in with your person to see if they have ideas for a legacy project and ask if they want to be a part of the process. Even if they simply sit at the table while you are sorting photos, this can be meaningful and important for them, and for you.

You might create a scrapbook or annotated photo album. You might write down the stories that your loved one had shared with you over the years. Or you might gather vignettes from people in your loved one's past. You could throw a party where everyone shares a memory, or you could take special pictures of your person with everyone that they love. Framing them, hanging them on the wall, and showing the finished product to your loved one would be a powerfully loving thing to do.

Is it Too Early to Think About a Legacy Project?

It's never too early to think about a legacy project.

I have written love letters to my husband and my girls that I keep in my underwear drawer, just in case. I want them to have letters to read and re-read in case I lose the opportunity to tell them how much I adore them and why.

I created treasure boxes for my girls a few Christmases ago. I wrote a heartfelt letter to each of them, then painted over the words. Then I cut up the pretty, painted paper into shapes, and decorated their boxes. The idea of the occasional loving word peeking through the paint makes me happy. I imagine them filling the boxes with things that make them feel special. Over the years I have also created multimedia art pieces for them and written them each a personalized poem.

It is never too early to create a legacy project.

QUESTION TO PONDER

What legacy would you like to leave?

FAMILY DISCUSSION QUESTION

Who in the family would like to work on a legacy project?

EXERCISE

Create a legacy project for yourself or with your loved one.

CHAPTER 16

Lean into Love

My father-in-law was murdered.

We found out on Christmas day. He was a widower with two sons, and my husband and his brother were in shock. They didn't feel able to cope with the endless complicated details associated with a violent death while they were grieving and processing this tragic family event, so I offered to take it on.

My husband seemed frozen. His dad's house had to be sold and someone had to manage the financial affairs and deal with the detectives. I did it with the help of kind friends, but it was brutal and I was a mess. I held it together when my girls were home, and then cried the whole time they were at school. I paced through the house and I couldn't sleep. It was surreal to see our family's story on the news, and the chaos went on for months. I was struggling, but I wanted to spare my husband because his grief and pain were exponentially more profound than mine. I did what had to be done.

This is love.

Jeffrey's parents would have given their own lives to save his. He was in his twenties and battling a brutal cancer that had robbed him of his strength, his speech, and his dreams. They drove hundreds of hours over multiple years to get him the best possible medical care, they visited countless rehabilitation specialists, and they tried to create normalcy out of chaos so Jeffrey could imagine a future for himself. Although their grief threatened to overwhelm them every minute of every day, they showed up for Jeffrey anyway, so he'd have a strong mom and dad to lean on.

This is love.

Sheila visited her mom, Millie, every day. Millie had dementia and it was becoming clear that she wouldn't be able to live alone for long. Sheila's siblings had differing opinions about what to do, and the differences in their coping styles made compromise challenging and sticky. Sheila hated watching her beloved mother become someone unrecognizable, and she hated arguing with her siblings. But she showed up every day to make her mom lunch, listen to stories that she'd heard before, and negotiate with her brothers and sisters.

This is love.

George hadn't showered for days. He had been in the ICU at his wife's bedside, watching her rhythmic, machine-controlled breaths and listening to a cacophony of beeps and alarms. He was both bored and terrified, and when the doctors came into her room his heart pounded and he felt light-headed. He was stone faced when they told him that she would never recover, and he held her hand when they turned off the breathing machine that had been keeping her alive.

This is love.

Carmen shaved her sister Donna's head when her hair fell out in chunks. When Donna felt like puking, Carmen brought her crackers, lukewarm soup, and some marijuana that she had gotten from her son. She kept people away when Donna just wanted to be left alone and updated all the key family and friends so they would know how things were going. She tried to match Donna's mood and could go from perky and hopeful to pragmatic or deep, depending on what Donna needed. She celebrated when the news was great and went into action and support mode when it wasn't.

This is love.

Ben, a physician, supported his wife, Amy, through an excruciating and mysterious illness. It tortured him that he couldn't fix her suffering. He scoured the medical literature for clues to a diagnosis and found specialists for her who were the best of the best. For many months, nothing helped. The more she suffered, the more anxious and distraught he became. In addition to supporting his wife in every way he could think of, Ben actively attended to his own well-being so he could continue to be there for Amy.

This is love.

Lana was tired of being a caregiver. She was depleted and exhausted and cranky. She wished that she were the kind of person who could be gracious and grateful and see caregiving as a privilege. She wasn't. Sometimes she wanted to run away, but she didn't. She showed up every day and did what had to be done.

This is love.

Microwaving dinner is love. Throwing in a load of laundry is love. Cleaning your loved one's rear end is love. Reading this book is love.

Showing up is love.

You'll have times when you are loving and kind and grateful. And then you'll have times when you are grumpy, exhausted, and impatient. This is normal. It happens to all caregivers. Just keep showing up.

Caring for someone who is ill is hard. Really hard. It *can* be sweet, of course, but it can also be brutal. It can make you feel incompetent, impotent, and mean. You may not be living up to your idealized version of the caregiver that you thought you'd be. You may not even recognize the person that you've become.

But you are doing your best, and your best is enough.

You are enough.

Life is messy and confusing, and you never know what the heck is going to happen next. Despite all your attempts to fix or control your situation, you really can't know what kind of tomorrow you'll get.

So, what are we supposed to do with this kind of mess?

Just keep showing up.

Every day, bring the best self that you can muster and do the best that you can to show love to someone else, show love to yourself, or at least wipe the crumbs off the counter.

This is the life we get.

We don't get to choose all the details, but we do get to choose how we carry ourselves through the story.

Sometimes we might shrivel and fold inwards, other times we might stride forward with our spine straight and our shoulders back. And every now and then, even sometimes in the midst of chaos or sadness or fear, we might turn our face to the sun and stretch our fingers to the sky.

Don't live the grayed-out version of life. Live the one that is full of color and nuance and the smell of sizzling garlic. Cry all the tears and feel all the feels. Pet the puppies and walk in the rain.

Just feel the whole thing. Allow both the love and the grief to touch your heart.

My wish for you is that you allow yourself to bathe in the mystery and awe of it all.

Epilogue

While I was writing this book, three souls who were important to me left this Earth. Two human, one canine. All three died in the span of two weeks. As I was writing about communication, I was communicating with my own family, talking to palliative care doctors, and making end-of-life decisions for my beloved fourteen-year-old dog.

I wrote and I cried. I cried and I wrote.

The humans were far too young to be leaving this earth, and the dog was so integrated into our family that my daughters both traveled home to say goodbye.

That time, rough as it was, reminded me that in writing this book I have been talking to myself as much as I have been talking to you. There is not a teacher and a student. We are all students, and we are all teachers.

Because this is the human condition.

Over the years, three of my dear friends have faced breast cancer and one of my cousins died suddenly in his thirties.

Everyone has stories like these.

Everyone has these stories because illness is a part of life.

Doctors try to banish it with IVs and scalpels and pills. Sometimes it works, but not always.

Coping with this part of life takes courage.

Several of my patients, as they got close to death, reported seeing deceased loved ones at their bedside. No one else could see these visitors, but to the patients they were clearly real. I have no idea what this is, but it happens often enough that I'm pretty sure it's something.

After my father-in-law died, he visited me several times. I'm not sure I believed in that sort of thing until I experienced it. But I certainly believe it now.

I don't know why some people get better and others don't. I don't know how people who have died can visit people who are living.

All I know is that we are in this together.

It is all a mystery, isn't it?

Acknowledgements

I am immensely grateful to Sarah Brown and Geoffrey Berwind, who made me believe that I could write a book and then helped me to birth it. Without them it would still be a half-done file on my computer.

Thank you to Cristina Smith, Valerie Costa, Christy Day, and Steve Scholl for molding my imperfect draft into an actual book that was ready for the world. Thank you to everyone who gave feedback about the cover, listened to my writing plans over coffee, and strategized with me about how to get this book into the hands of more people who could benefit from it.

Thank you to all of my patients, and their families, who taught me to be a more thoughtful, wise, skilled, and open-hearted doctor.

I am beyond grateful to my husband, Tony, who supported me (and brought me water and coffee) as I spent hour after hour in my special writing chair. Thank you to my friends and first readers who read my chapters and gave honest, wise, and thoughtful feedback. You absolutely made the book better.

Thank you to my beloved daughters who encouraged me to grow as a person and explore the experience of writing a book. Watching you stretch into ever-expanding versions of yourselves ignited my desire to try something new.

And deepest thanks to my tiny, fuzzy writing buddy, Coco. Thanks for taking me most of the way home.

About the Author

DELIA CHIARAMONTE, MD, MS is an experienced integrative palliative medicine physician and medical educator. She is the founder of the Integrative Palliative Institute and host of *The Integrative Palliative Podcast*. As a thought leader in the field of integrative palliative medicine, she specializes in whole-person care for families facing serious illness, using all the tools that work. As a person who has been a caregiver, Dr. Chiaramonte understands, from the inside, the fear, stress, and overwhelm that people face when someone they love is unwell.

Dr. Chiaramonte is the former associate director and director of education for the University of Maryland Medical School's Center for Integrative Medicine and the former division chief of integrative palliative medicine at Greater Baltimore Medical Center/Gilchrist. She has been voted a "Top Doctor" by her peers and won awards for teaching excellence. As a sought-after lecturer, she has been invited to teach at organizations such as Johns Hopkins Hospital, the University of San Francisco Medical School, the University of Maryland Graduate School, and School of Pharmacy and The American College of Rheumatology. She has published chapters in the textbooks *Practical Management of Pain* and *Families in the Intensive Care Unit* and serves as an executive editor for McGraw Hill Education. She is an adjunct assistant professor at the University of Maryland, Baltimore.

Dr. Chiaramonte is a dynamic and engaging keynote speaker, and she is **available for speaking engagements and media interviews.** To schedule Dr. Chiaramonte for an interview or speaking engagement, visit www.DrChiaramonte.com. She offers a **companion toolkit to this book for families facing serious illness.** Information about this program is available at www.CopingCourageously.com.

She "fills her cup" by drinking coffee with her grown daughters, reading, going for walks with friends, and creating multi-media art. She lives in Maryland with her husband and her brand-new rescue dog, Sadie.

www.CopingCourageously.com

Free Offers

The Essential Caregiving Checklist:
What You Need to Do If Someone You Love is Ill

If someone you love is sick, you may feel overwhelmed, exhausted, and unsure. There are so many details and things to worry about that it can be hard to know what to focus on. As an integrative palliative care physician who has cared for many families just like you, I've created a practical checklist to guide you.

This helpful guide provides key steps to help your family effectively navigate this challenging time.

You can find the free Essential Caregiving Checklist at:
www.CopingSupport.com

For Physicians and Clinicians:
How to Support Families Who Are Facing Serious Illness

If you are a physician, nurse practitioner, physician assistant, social worker, chaplain, or other healthcare clinician, you want to support your patients or clients (and their families) as they face serious illness, but you may not know exactly what to say or how best to help.

As an integrative palliative care physician, I know just how tough this can be. I've created an integrative symptom management guide to help you deliver the best possible care to your seriously ill patients.

It includes effective and simple ways to care for yourself too, because if you get depleted you can't be the empathetic clinician that you want to be. If you're not at your best, nobody wins.

Expanding your toolbox to include an evidence-supported integrative approach is the best way to care for your patients, their families, and yourself.

Get your helpful clinician guide at:
www.CopingSupport.com